NEURAL STEM CELL RESEARCH

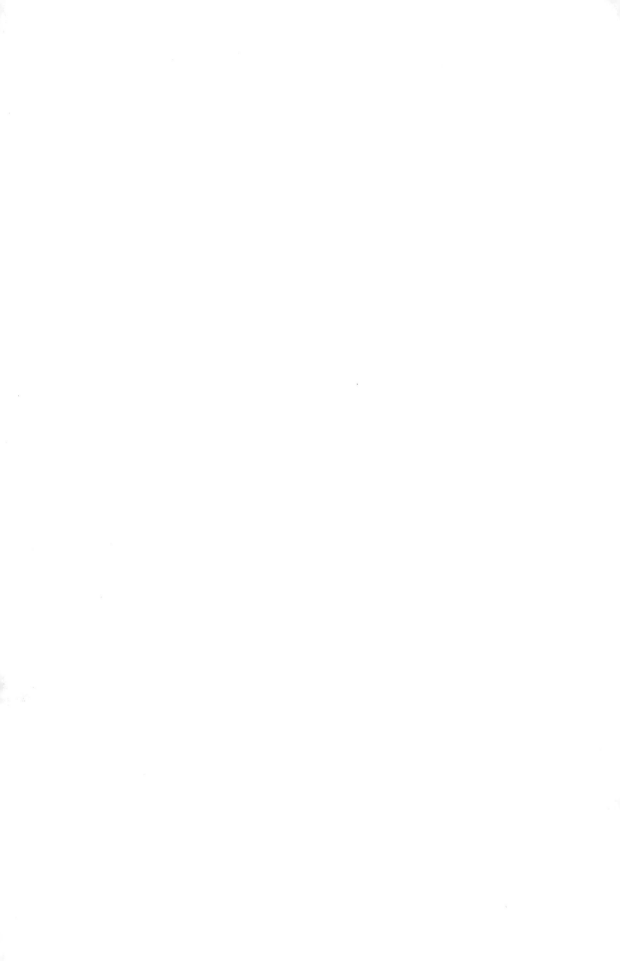

NEURAL STEM CELL RESEARCH

ERIC V. GRIER
EDITOR

Nova Science Publishers, Inc.
New York

NOTICE TO THE READER

The Publisher has taken reasonable care in the preparation of this book, but makes no expressed or implied warranty of any kind and assumes no responsibility for any errors or omissions. No liability is assumed for incidental or consequential damages in connection with or arising out of information contained in this book. The Publisher shall not be liable for any special, consequential, or exemplary damages resulting, in whole or in part, from the readers' use of, or reliance upon, this material.

This publication is designed to provide accurate and authoritative information with regard to the subject matter covered herein. It is sold with the clear understanding that the Publisher is not engaged in rendering legal or any other professional services. If legal or any other expert assistance is required, the services of a competent person should be sought. FROM A DECLARATION OF PARTICIPANTS JOINTLY ADOPTED BY A COMMITTEE OF THE AMERICAN BAR ASSOCIATION AND A COMMITTEE OF PUBLISHERS.

Library of Congress Cataloging-in-Publication Data
Neural stem cell research / Erik V. Grier, editor.
    p. ; cm.
 Includes bibliographical references and index.
 ISBN 1-59454-846-3
 1. Neural stem cells. 2. Neural stem cells--Transplantation. 3. Nervous system--Regeneration.
 [DNLM: 1. Neurons--physiology. 2. Stem Cells--physiology. 3. Biomedical Research.
4. Models, Neurological. 5. Nerve Regeneration. 6. Stem Cell Transplantation. WL 102.5
N492415 2006] I. Greer, Erik V.

QP356.25.N463 2006
612.6'4018--dc22
2005033511

Published by Nova Science Publishers, Inc. ✦ New York

CONTENTS

PREFACE

Among the many applications of stem cell research are nervous system diseases, diabetes, heart disease, autoimmune diseases as well as Parkinson's disease, end-stage kidney disease, liver failure, cancer, spinal cord injury, multiple sclerosis, Parkinson's disease, and Alzheimer's disease. Stem cells are self-renewing, unspecialized cells that can give rise to multiple types all of specialized cells of the body. Stem cell research also involves complex ethical and legal considerations since they involve adult, fetal tissue and embryonic sources. This new book brings together leading research from throughout the world in this frontier field.

Research on stem cell transplantation as potential therapy for neurodegenerative disorders has increased dramatically in the last 5 years. However, the mechanism whereby transplanted cells might integrate 'appropriately' throughout the mammalian nervous system is still poorly understood. Recent studies have demonstrated that transplanted neural stem cells are capable of engrafting in a cytoarchitecturally and developmentally appropriate manner within the normal and abnormal central nervous system (CNS) following transplantation. Furthermore, studies have shown that the transplanted neural stem cells are capable of migrating to areas of the CNS affected by disease or injury; that is, these transplanted cells have the ability to 'hone in' on pathology, even over great distances. Given these recent reports, Teresita L. Briones' discussion in *Interactions between Transplanted Neural Stem Cells and Host Tissue: A Two-Way Street* will include the phenomenon of how the host CNS environment instructs and influence the fate of transplanted neural stem cells migrating to areas of pathology and assuming the phenotype(s) of host cells that are affected by disease or injury. Moreover, the emerging data on the capability of transplanted cells to instruct and alter the fate of host CNS tissue will also be covered in this chapter. The growing evidence to support the notion that donor neural stem cells and host tissue communicate in a reciprocal fashion will also be discussed. For example, while it has been demonstrated that a given host CNS environment is instructive of donor stem cells, influencing their migration and differentiation patterns, the donor neural stem cells are apparently equally capable of manipulating their milieu. However, the signals generated by neural stem cells to communicate with the host tissue have yet to be identified but it is speculated that molecules such as growth factors, cell adhesion molecules, cytokines and chemokines are involved. This continuously evolving understanding of how the donor neural stem cells are interacting with host tissue in a regenerative or restorative manner will be the main focus of this chapter.

In situ, neural stem cells are located in a niche that consists of a restricted set of cell types and contains a specialised microenvironment composed of soluble factors, membrane-bound molecules and extracellular matrix components. The roles of extracellular matrix (ECM) molecules in the development, maintenance and plasticity of the central nervous system have been the subject of increasing study. The in vivo expression profile of these molecules, notably in and leading out of the germinal zones, especially the subventricular zone, has given clues as to their influence on a range of developmental processes, including proliferation, migration, survival, and process outgrowth. In vitro studies on primary cell cultures and neural stem cell-derived neurospheres have confirmed cell-type specific effects of ECM molecules such as the glycoprotein, Tenascin-C, the proteoglycan, phosphacan, and of post-translational carbohydrate modifications on ECM and cell adhesion molecules, such as PSA, Lewis-X and HNK-1. Recent data derived from analysis of transgenic knockout mice is further contributing to an understanding of the roles of these ECM molecules in CNS development and regeneration. Most notably, Tenascin-C has now been shown to alter the responsiveness of neural stem cells and stem-cell derived precursors to several growth factors, including bFGF, BMP-4, and PDGF, thereby affecting the generation of a stem cell niche within the subventricular zone by acting to orchestrate growth factor signalling and the rate of neural stem cell development. The nature of these effects on neural stem cells and oligodendrocyte precursor cell behaviour is considered in more detail in *Roles of Extracellular Matrix Molecules in Neural Stem Cell Development and the Example of Tenascin-C* by Jeremy Garwood.

Neural stem cells can be isolated from various regions of the adult brain, including the regions with spontaneous neurogenesis, i. e. the dentate gyrus of the hippocampus, and the subventricular zone. With regard to proliferation and differentiation, the properties of these adult neural stem and progenitor cells have been defined as (i) postnatal cells in the adult brain capable of cell division, (ii) self-renewing the stem cell precursor pool, and (iii) giving rise to differentiated cells of the neural, astrocytic, and oligodendrocytic lineage. Whereas their proliferative activity and differentiation potential has been well characterized, a generally accepted cellular marker for the neural stem and progenitor cell has not yet been established. In this article, efforts are described to specify such markers.

Most of the promising candidates for neural stem cell markers such as nestin, doublecortin, Musashi-1, or Mcm2, are not exclusively expressed in neural stem cells, or when expressed, this happens only during a short time period of development. Consequently, the search for specific markers has been expanded to new high-throughput techniques based on genomic, transcriptomic, or proteomic screening of embryonic and adult neural stem cells.

In *Towards a Molecular Signature of Neural Stem Cells*, Martin H. Maurer and Wolfgang Kuschinsky discuss the use of the most prominent presumptive neural stem cell markers currently in use to identify these cells. The authors evaluate their expression with regard to time and specificity, and summarize the current standard protocols for neural stem cell staining. In the second section of this chapter, they compare gene expression patterns of neural stem cells, which exist on the genome or transcriptome level, with gene expression patterns of other stem cells. In the third section of the chapter, the current literature on stem cell proteomics is reviewed. Protein inventories of neural stem cells at different times of development and different status of differentiation have been created as a basis of protein expression analysis. Now, these inventories are increasingly used for differential protein expression studies.

Maurer and Kuschinsky summarize the pros and cons of the current stem cell markers and comment on large-scale genomic, transcriptomic, and proteomic approaches for the search of a stem cell specific expression pattern. They conclude that agreement on the cellular markers of neural stem cells is still lacking.

Neural stem cells (NSCs) research has been characterized by an extraordinary expansion over the past few years also in view of new possible therapies for neurodegenerative diseases. The use of neural stem-based cell therapy to overcome the scarce potential repair capacity of an injured/diseased brain constitutes one of the more responsible cues that NSCs's research has to deal with. Many studies have focused on the use of NSCs for grafting specific neural cell types into effected areas, in a great number of animal models of neurodegenerative diseases such as Alzheimer disease's (AD) (Jin et al., 2004), Parkinson disease's (PD) (Sanchez-Pernaute et al., 2005; Sorensen et al., 2005), multiple sclerosis (MS) (Pluchino et al., 2003), spinal cord injury (Okano et al., 2002) and stroke (Haas et al., 2005).

In order to unveil the proliferative and differentiative potential of NSCs and their use for cell replacement therapeutic purposes, it is of extreme importance: i) to identify genes responsible for proliferation and/or differentiation regulation of NSCs and to know how they act; ii) to understand the mechanisms that regulate NSCs biological and physiological functions; iii) to study key molecules capable of enhancing the potential of endogenous NSCs to proliferate and differentiate into specific cell phenotypes to achieve structural and functional brain repair. In order to pursue these goals, *in vivo* and *in vitro* models are being used so far. Although *in vivo* models reflect in a more realistic fashion the environment of a diseased brain, due to the complexity of the mechanisms underlying neurodegenerative diseases, simplified *in vitro* approaches are often useful to investigate many fundamental biological processes that take part in these pathologies.

In our recent work, M. Fernández, M. Paradisi, L. Giardino and L. Calzà have attempted to at least partially overcome limitations intrinsic to both *in vivo* and *in vitro* approaches for NSCs understanding, focusing on the *in vitro* study of properties of neurospheres generated from brains of rats affected by experimental pathologies and pharmacologically treated. "Neurospheres" are heterogeneous aggregates of cells, also including NSCs, which can be obtained and expanded from the subventricular zone in the forebrain of adult animals (Pevny and Rao, 2003). We focused in particular on the possible role of endogenous NSCs and oligodendrocyte precursors in the re-myelination capability of the mature central nervous system (CNS). It is in fact well known that remyelination is possibly the only true, robust repair capability of the mature CNS, due to the large number of oligodendrocyte precursor cells (OPCs) which are widely disseminated in the white and grey matter (Chen et al., 2002). However, for unknown reason, this capability is lost or defective in a percentage of patients affected by MS, the most diffuse demyelinating disease (Lubetzki et al., 2005), thus leading to the axonal and neuronal damage which is responsible for chronic disabilities (Bruck and Stadelmann, 2005; D'Intino et al., 2005). Their previous *in vivo* work has demonstrated that NSCs in the SVZ are highly susceptible to the microenvironmental conditions observed in the inflammatory phase of the inflammatory demyelinating disease experimental allergic encephalomyelitis (EAE), which is the most widely used model for MS (Calzà et al., 1998, 2004), whereas other lesions, which includes a low inflammatory response, inhibits rather than stimulates proliferation rate in the SVZ (Calzà et al., 2004). They have also proved that the *in vivo* administration of thyroid hormone (TH), which is the key signal for oligodendrocyte generation during CNS development, regulates cell proliferation in the SVZ and favours oligodendrocyte generation and maturation (Calzà et al., 2002; Fernández et al., 2004; Calzà et al., 2005). The authors have proved that EAE induces extensive proliferation of OPCs (NG2-, A2B5- PDGF alfa R-expressing cells) and that administration of TH is able to promote faster and complete myelination. Moreover, expression of cell cycle-associated markers in NSCs in the SVZ, which also proliferate actively in the acute phase of EAE (e.g. under inflammatory stimuli), significantly decreases in EAE rats treated with TH during a precise time-window corresponding to intense proliferation.

The authors have contributed as well to the hypothesis that oligodendrocyte development and myelination are under TH control not only during development, but also in the adult life, possibly affecting re-myelination capability of the mature CNS (Fernández et al., 2004).

In *To Know Neural Stem Properties from Diseased Brains: A Critical Step for Brain Repair*, M. Fernández et al. present the protocols that we routinely use in the lab for standardization and quantification of neurosphere production from the adult rat brain, for characterization of derived cells and application on diseased brains. All the materials used and the procedures followed have been described in great detail in Appendix 1 and Appendix 2, respectively, in this chapter.

Taurine is a β-amino acid that serves important functions in mammalian brain development. However, no data are available about its distribution and possible roles in neural precursors from a non-retinal origin. Neural stem cells (NSC) with self-renewal and multilineage potential are an important tool to study the signals involved in the regulation of brain development. Eulalia Bazán, Antonio S. Herranz, Diana Reimers, Maria V.T. Lobo, Carolina Redondo, Miguel A. López-Toledano, Rafael Gonzalo-Gobernado, Maria J. Asensio and Raquel Alonso investigate the role played by taurine during the differentiation of NSC from fetal rat striatum *Neural Stem Cells and Taurine*. Taurine content was analyzed in the cultures by HPLC at different times post-plating. Between 2 and 24 hours taurine was detected at a basal value of 7 nmol/mg protein. As cells were maintained in culture, this value increased to reach 40 nmol/mg protein at 10 days post-plating. Taurine immunoreactivity was found in nestin, A2B5, β-tubulin III and O1 positive cells. The addition for 1 to 3 days of 2 mM taurine to recently seeded neurospheres increased its intracellular content by 28 fold, and high taurine levels were maintained even 7 days after taurine withdrawal. By contrast, cultures treated with 2 mM of the high-affinity taurine transporter inhibitor guanidinoethanesulfonic acid (GES) showed a sharp decrease in taurine content. When taurine was applied in combination with GES, taurine levels were significantly higher than those observed after GES treatment. Taurine treatment did not affect the relative amount of neurons and oligodendrocytes in the cultures, but promoted the differentiation of O1-positive cells that showed an increase in the length and number of their processes. We conclude that NSC develop specific taurine uptake mechanisms at early stages differentiation. Since taurine was not present in the feeding medium, we suggest that NSC and their progeny have the machinery for taurine synthesis. Present results also indicate that taurine might influence the development of NSC oligodendroglial progeny.

Retrovirus vectors suffer severe gene silencing in stem cells that hampers their use in stem cell gene therapy. Transduced retrovirus vector can be completely silenced, or dynamically silenced in a subset of cells resulting in variegation. Expressing retrovirus also can be extinguished during stem cell differentiation. Multiple epigenetic modifications including histone modifications and DNA methylation are functionally involved in establishing and maintaining retrovirus silencing via the formation of silent chromatin. Shuyuan Yao and James Ellis propose a model is that the balance of epigenetic effects at the integration site and retroviral silencer elements on the vectors determines the decision to be silent, variegated or expressing in stem cells in *Retrovirus Vector Silencing in Stem Cells*. Silencing resistant retrovirus vectors have been developed by removal of these silencer elements, and silencing in stem cells may ultimately be blocked using appropriate insulator elements.

Advances in fluorescent probing and microscopic imaging technology provide important tools for biology and medicine research in studying the structures and functions of cells and molecules. Such studies require the processing and analysis of huge amounts of image data, and manual image analysis is very time consuming, thus costly, and also potentially inaccurate and poorly reproducible. Stages of an automated cellular imaging analysis consist of segmentation, feature extraction, classification, and tracking of individual cells in a dynamic cellular population. Image classification of cell phases in a fully automatic manner presents the most difficult task of such analysis. Tuan D. Pham, Dat T. Tran, Xiaobo Zhou and Stephen T.C. Wong are interested in applying several advanced computational, probabilistic, and fuzzy-set methods for the computerized classification of cell nuclei in different mitotic phases in *Classification of Cell Phases in Time-Lapse Images by Vector Quantization and Markov Models*. They tested several proposed computational procedures with real image sequences recorded over a period of twenty-four hours at every fifteen minutes with a time-lapse fluorescence microscopy. The experimental results have shown that the proposed methods are effective and has potential for higher performance with better cellular feature extraction strategy.

In: Neural Stem Cell Research
Editor: Eric V. Grier, pp. 1-26

ISBN: 1-59454-846-3
© 2006 Nova Science Publishers, Inc.

Chapter 1

INTERACTIONS BETWEEN TRANSPLANTED NEURAL STEM CELLS AND HOST TISSUE: A TWO-WAY STREET

Teresita L. Briones[*]

Department of Medical-Surgical Nursing
University of Illinois at Chicago

Abstract

Research on stem cell transplantation as potential therapy for neurodegenerative disorders has increased dramatically in the last 5 years. However, the mechanism whereby transplanted cells might integrate 'appropriately' throughout the mammalian nervous system is still poorly understood. Recent studies have demonstrated that transplanted neural stem cells are capable of engrafting in a cytoarchitecturally and developmentally appropriate manner within the normal and abnormal central nervous system (CNS) following transplantation. Furthermore, studies have shown that the transplanted neural stem cells are capable of migrating to areas of the CNS affected by disease or injury; that is, these transplanted cells have the ability to 'hone in' on pathology, even over great distances. Given these recent reports, discussion on this chapter will include the phenomenon of how the host CNS environment instructs and influence the fate of transplanted neural stem cells migrating to areas of pathology and assuming the phenotype(s) of host cells that are affected by disease or injury. Moreover, the emerging data on the capability of transplanted cells to instruct and alter the fate of host CNS tissue will also be covered in this chapter. The growing evidence to support the notion that donor neural stem cells and host tissue communicate in a reciprocal fashion will also be discussed. For example, while it has been demonstrated that a given host CNS environment is instructive of donor stem cells, influencing their migration and differentiation patterns, the donor neural stem cells are apparently equally capable of

---

[*] Phone: (312) 355-3142,Fax: (312) 996-4979,Email: tbriones@uic.edu; Correspondence: Teresita L. Briones, Ph.D.,University of Illinois at Chicago, 845 S. Damen Ave., M/C 802, Rm 750,Chicago, IL 60612

manipulating their milieu. However, the signals generated by neural stem cells to communicate with the host tissue have yet to be identified but it is speculated that molecules such as growth factors, cell adhesion molecules, cytokines and chemokines are involved. This continuously evolving understanding of how the donor neural stem cells are interacting with host tissue in a regenerative or restorative manner will be the main focus of this chapter.

Introduction

The mammalian central nervous system (CNS) is incredibly complex and possesses only a limited ability to recover from injury. These characteristics of the CNS have made therapeutic management of neurological disorders very difficult. The limited inherent capability of the CNS to recover from insult is also the main reason why most research into brain and spinal cord injuries primarily focused on promoting axonal regeneration and reducing neuronal degeneration. Fortunately, the discovery of self-renewing stem cell populations within the fetal and adult brain has opened promising lines of investigation into the treatment of CNS disorders [1,2]. More recently, the potential of using stem cells as a tool to treat CNS disorders has gained increased attention because of encouraging results in neural transplantation research. The original intent to use neural grafts for CNS repair was to take advantage of the highly plastic characteristics of dividing cells residing in the germinal zones of the developing brain and spinal cord, and at the same time of the relatively higher immunologic tolerance of the CNS [3]. The possibility that the immature donor tissue might replace dysfunctional host cells or deliver missing substances into the impaired host tissue has generated new hope in developing therapies for the management of CNS disorders. Yet the current data, although promising still present some doubts on the effectiveness of cell replacement therapy as a cure for neurodegeneration or CNS injury. Some of the difficulties encountered in cell replacement therapy (e.g. poor cell survival and limited differentiation) may be attributed to the topographic maps in the CNS that are interrelated to one another in very specific ways. Thus, to replace damaged neural cells presents a problem that cannot be easily solved by 'just' delivering suitable cells that would survive and differentiate in the host environment – the common experimental approach used in cell replacement therapy. For grafted cells to become functional, it is necessary for the donor cells to establish appropriate afferent and efferent connections to maintain the specificity of the CNS topographic map. Consequently, it is important to understand the reciprocal signals generated by the donor and host cells to communicate with each other - the main focus of this review - so that successful regeneration can be facilitated.

Sources of Cells for Transplantation

Depending on the donor material, neural grafts have been proposed to facilitate morphologic and functional recovery of the recipient CNS by either: (1) replacing affected cell populations (or its structural components like myelin) and their connections, which can then lead to functional recovery, (2) delivering missing neuroactive molecules, such as enzymes and neurotransmitters, (3) providing a growth-permissive tissue "bridges" for host axonal regeneration and target-oriented guidance of growing axons, and (4) enhancing secretion of neurotrophic and other regeneration-promoting substances that supports the survival and growth of both graft and host cells. There are four main sources of cells for transplantation: neural tissue stem cells, embryonic stem cells, non-neuronal tissue cells, and immortalized cell lines.

Neural Tissue Stem Cells

Neural tissue cells (NSCs) have been identified in many areas of the developing mammalian brain, and also in specific regions of the adult CNS [1,4]. Such cells are easy to expand and have been demonstrated to differentiate into all three neural cell types - neurons, oligodendrocytes and astrocytes [5,6]. For instance, murine NSCs isolated from developing brain and spinal cord generated neurospheres, self-renewed and differentiated into neurons and glia. Subsequent transplantation of these neurospheres into the lateral ventricles of immunodeficient newborn NOD/SCID mice then showed engraftment, migration and region-specific neuronal differentiation on examination up to 7 months later [7]. When considering NSCs for cell replacement therapies, it is important to be cognizant of the fact that cells from different brain regions are not identical, displaying different growth characteristics, trophic factor requirements and restricted patterns of differentiation. In addition, these multipotent cells clearly differ in their potential according to the developmental stage at which they were isolated and the specific brain region from which they were isolated. Although the bulk of experimental data has been obtained using rodent NSCs, similar multipotent cells have been identified in humans.

The presence of NSCs are not exclusive to the developing or fetal brain as demonstrated by numerous pioneering studies that identified two distinct regions of the adult mammalian CNS that contain populations of NSCs [1,2,8]. The identified sites where NSCs are present in the adult brain are the: subgranular zone of the dentate gyrus [1] and the subventricular zone (SVZ) of the lateral ventricles [9]. It has also been shown that NSCs in the adult brain are not only present in the SVZ but also in the entire rostral extension, including the distal portion within the olfactory bulb [10]. Although these endogenous adult NSCs have been shown to proliferate, migrate to the olfactory bulb and hippocampus, and ultimately differentiate into mature neurons, their functionality is not clear. In an elegant study done that used a virus-based trans-synaptic neuronal tracing and *c-fos* mapping it was demonstrated that the endogenous adult NSCs upregulated the expression of *c-fos* proto-oncogene in the olfactory bulb in response to an odor-induced signal [6,11]. These results indicate that adult NSCs can differentiate into newly formed adult neurons and functionally integrate into the synaptic circuitry of the mature brain.

Adult NSCs can also be isolated from the adult human brain. Indeed, such cells have now been cultured from human cadavers up to 20 days after death [12]. Although adult NSCs demonstrate a high degree of plasticity, they are difficult to isolate, found in smaller numbers, have a more limited proliferative capacity, and seem to have a more restricted differentiation potential than their fetal counterparts [13].

Embryonic Stem Cells

Embryonic stem (ES) cells are obtained from the inner cell mass of the blastocyst of fetuses and can give rise to all tissues in the body, including those of the nervous system. ES cells are also multipotent, can be propagated *in vitro* and can be engineered to express therapeutic genes thus, provide the most promising alternative source of cells for transplant. When used for transplant, ES cells can migrate and differentiate into regionally appropriate cell types, and did not appear to interfere with normal brain development [14]. Initially, it has been reported that murine ES cells can be induced to express multiple neural phenotypes in culture using retinoic acid as the trigger for differentiation [15]. Following differentiation, it was found that the newly formed neurons were capable of generating action potentials and expressed numerous ion channels. In addition, others have reported that the ES cells expanded and differentiated into oligodendrocyte precursors and were able to effectively myelinate host axons in animal models of human myelin disease [16,17].

Other studies have demonstrated that ES cells transplanted following focal forebrain ischemic injury in adult rats, not only survived in the infarct area but also established connections to the surrounding brain regions, with a resulting improvement in motor function [18-20], spatial learning, and memory [21,22]. Moreover, clinical trials of patients with Parkinson's disease that received ES cell grafts into the striatum showed that the grafted cells were spontaneously active and was able to restore dopamine release to near-normal levels with symptomatic improvement [23,24]. However, cell-based therapy in humans using ES cells has mixed results since in a recent clinical trial in Denver and New York showed that 15% of grafted patients developed unacceptable dyskinesias [23]. Immune rejection and subsequent failure of the graft can also be a problem associated with ES cell therapy, particularly in human clinical trials.

The major concern in using ES cells is its limited supply and the small number of neurons that can be generated and become available for transplant [13]. However, this problem may be partially overcome by *in vitro* expansion as demonstrated in a study wherein human ES cell isolated from the forebrain were expanded for up to a year in culture using epithelial growth factor (EGF), fibroblast growth factor (FGF), and leukemia inhibitory factor (LIF) [25]. Additionally, prolonged culture did not profoundly affect the potential of these expanded ES cells, and indeed injection of these cell lines into the developing rat brain showed extensive migration and integration [26]. Others have confirmed these findings and have shown that enriched neural precursors from human ES cells can incorporate into brain tissue and differentiate *in vivo* [27,28]. When these expanded human ES cells were transplanted into the lateral ventricles of newborn mice, migration to multiple brain regions was observed, followed by differentiation into cells with mature neuronal and astrocytic phenotypes but no mature oligodendrocytes were seen. In addition, embryonic day 12 (E12) cells propagated in culture have also been shown to retain the capacity to differentiate into dopaminergic neurons and to improve outcome in a rat model of Parkinson's disease [29]. These studies demonstrating the success of ES cell grafts *in vivo* has led to further work in other injury models to see whether transplanted cells can integrate and functionally improve outcome in different CNS injuries. Although present results on neural grafting using ES cells are encouraging, it is clear that challenges remain notwithstanding the highly controversial nature of the source of these cells.

Non-Neuronal Tissue Cells

To circumvent the ethical issues concerning the use of ES cells for transplantation, a growing number of studies suggest that non-neural cell types (e.g. bone marrow cells) can be propagated and differentiated into neural lineages. Much of this work is controversial but if useful neural cells could be obtained from this source, it would avoid the ethical problems associated with the use of ES cells, and the practical issues of deriving cells from post-mortem brains. The early *in vivo* experimental data using non-neuronal cells was based on bone marrow transplantation (BMT) studies in lethally irradiated mice [30]. More recently, it has been shown that bone marrow-derived cells transplanted into the adult rat striatum after cerebral ischemia resulted in the amelioration of ischemia-induced neurological deficits [31]. There are now several published protocols for directing bone marrow stromal cells to neural lineages using different approaches that can range from using chemical demethylating or reducing agents, to retinoids and use of more physiological growth factors [32]. The successful generation of neural cells from blood could either be due to the presence of a minute subpopulation of highly pluripotent cells in the marrow, or explained by the reprogramming (trans- or dedifferentiation) of an already committed blood progenitor. Blood or bone marrow would be an ethically acceptable and easily accessible source of cells for neural replacement, although research in this area is still at an early stage and the findings are controversial.

Immortalized Cell Lines

Another alternative to ES cells comes in the form of immortalized cell lines. A pioneering study that used an exogenous cell line for regeneration in areas of the CNS was done in a rat model of stroke [33]. The cells used in that study was derived from a teratocarcinoma cell line, Ntera 2/cl.D1 (NT2), expanded in cell culture, and differentiated into pure postmitotic human neuronal cells following treatment with retinoic acid. Specifically, using the middle cerebral artery (MCA) occlusion model of stroke in rats, injection of the immortalized cells into the area of ischemia resulted in a partial restoration of behavioral and motor function [34]. Furthermore, follow-up study at 14 months showed no toxicity or tumor formation in the animals that received the graft [33]. Thereafter, a clinical trial that included 12 patients with basal ganglia stroke onset ranging from 6 months to 6 years received stereotactic injections of human teratocarcinoma (hNT) cells into their ischemic brain regions [35]. Results of this clinical trial showed an increase in the European Stroke Scale scores in patients that received the graft, thereby demonstrating that neuronal cell transplantation may be a therapeutic option for stroke patients with motor deficits. Further, using serial metabolic brain imaging with [^{18}F]fluorodeoxyglucose positron emission tomography that was obtained both before and after neural transplantation, patients that received the graft showed a 10% increase in functional activity at 6 months, with a return to baseline at 12 months. Although the immortalized cell lines showed promise as evident in these studies, they are not true stem cells and have been criticized for the difficulty in generating them especially for large-scale clinical use. Another criticism involving immortalized cell lines is that the initial reports lack convincing evidence on whether these cells actually integrated into the damaged parenchyma to form functionally significant neural network connections within the existing cytoarchitecture or how they might have contributed to behavioral recovery. Though a recent report using hNT cell lines transplanted into a rat model of complete spinal cord contusion with loss of motor evoked potentials addressed this concern [36]. In this spinal cord study, rats that underwent immediate and delayed (2 weeks after injury) transplantation of hNT showed significant functional recovery demonstrated by the return of motor evoked potentials and some degree of improvement in motor function.

Other immortalized cells lines that have been developed and tested are: C17.2 and CG4. The C17.2 immortalized cell line is derived from murine cerebellar external granular layer progenitor cells and transduced with a v-*myc* oncogene [37]. When transplanted into a targeted area of apoptotic neurodegeneration in the adult mouse neocortex, approximately 5% of the C17.2 cells differentiated into neurons and graft survival was seen up to 22 months [38]. In contrast, the CG4 immortalized cell line is an oligodendrocyte progenitor cells that has been used successfully for demyelinating diseases. For instance, a number of studies have demonstrated that CG4 transplantation into the spinal cord of rats with experimental autoimmune encephalomyelitis (EAE) survived for long periods of time, migrated as far as 6 cm from the site of injection, and repopulated areas of demyelination [39,40]. These studies suggest that immortalized cell lines may represent an additional source of exogenous cells to participate in neural repair involving CNS disorders. There are, however, considerable fears that use of immortalized cell lines may increase the incidence of tumorigenesis and that they may not be able to replace the wide variety of cell types lost after CNS injury which makes their clinical use limited.

Evidence of Graft/Host Communication Following Neural Transplantation

Over a decade ago, it was demonstrated that grafting fetal neural tissue induce plasticity in the host brain resulting in the repair of damaged neurons in a manner that was different from that seen in spontaneous CNS recovery [41]. This was evident in an earlier study in neural transplantation wherein primary neural tissue from the fetal mouse (embryonic day 14, E14) neopallium was transplanted into the mechanically damaged barrel field area of primary somatosensory cortex of juvenile mice [42]. In this study, two co-isogenic mouse strains were used so that donor cells could be easily and unambiguously identified from host cells by allelic differences in their Thy-1 antigen (cell surface marker for neural cells). Results from this study showed that one month after transplantation the lesion cavity in 70-80% of mice that received the grafted cells appeared to become "filled" by relatively well-organized cortical tissue that even presented cellular arrangements reminiscent of barrels and displayed some degree of electrical activity. In comparison, the barrel field lesion in mice that did not receive the grafted cells remained unaltered or in some instances grew even larger. Surprisingly, anti Thy-1 immunohistochemistry demonstrated that virtually all transplant-induced regenerated tissue was of host origin in over 50% of the animals. These results were later validated using a xenotransplantation paradigm (transplantation between different species) wherein mouse tissue was transplanted into lesioned cat CNS [43]. Specifically, neural tissue from fetal embryonic (E14) mouse neopallium was transplanted into the primary visual cortical lesion of 1-month-old kittens and results similar to the earlier study were seen. However, the percentage of successful xenografting was lower than that of the previous allografts (grafts between individuals within the same species). To examine whether de novo neurogenesis could explain the results seen in these studies, barrel field lesioned mice received either tritiated thymidine ($[^3H]T$) or bromodeoxyuridine (BrdU) which are nucleotide analogs that label dividing cells during the S-phase of the cell cycle [43]. The investigators found that the majority of ($[^3H]T$)- and BrdU-labeled host cells to be of glial and endothelial origin, although no significant gliosis or glial scar was evident . Because limited endogenous neurogenesis was seen in this study, it was not sufficient to account for the substantial tissue recovery seen. Thus, other mechanisms such as "remodeling" of surrounding tissue by existing postmitotic cells as well as prevention of necrosis and secondary host cell death in the vicinity of the cavity may explain the graft/host interaction that led to the enhanced plasticity seen in the previous studies [44].

Others have also reported a similar graft-dependent regeneration in the injured brain. Using bilateral parietal cortex lesion in rats, others have found that primary fetal neural tissue grafted unilaterally influenced neuronal regeneration in the contralateral non-transplanted cavity wherein the lesion became smaller as compared to the non-grafted lesioned controls [45]. More recently, graft/host interactions during brain development were examined where human NSCs were grafted *in utero* into the ventricles of a midgestation non-human primate brain [8]. Results from this study showed that the donor cells not only survived the xenotransplantation, but also integrated into the host brain. Evidence of this integration was seen when the grafted cells entered the subventricular zone, interdigitated with the endogenous NSCs, and together both host and donor cells subdivided into different phenotype in the developing brain. This "teamwork" of donor and host NSCs seen during brain development was reflected in a prevalent morphogenetic scenario. That is, many of the NSCs migrated out of the subventricular zone and started to differentiate into various types of neural cells, while other subpopulations of donor and host NSCs remained undifferentiated and formed quiescent pools of multipotent cells, possibly for later use during ontogeny or maintenance of CNS homeostasis. Based on the observations of graft-induced host plasticity in the developing and injured brain, it is likely that reciprocal communication between graft and host cells is multifaceted [44]. Other indications of graft/host communication have been demonstrated in the aged brain and in CNS pathologies due to trauma or genetic disorders.

Graft/Host Communication in the Aged Brain

The slow disintegration of neural function associated with aging provides an ideal opportunity to examine the reciprocal communication between the graft and host brain in an environment *not* confounded by excessive necrosis, excitotoxicity, anoxia, or trauma. Since dopaminergic neurons are typically compromised in advanced age, the study used systemic injection of MPTP (1-methyl-4-phenyl-1,2,3,6-tetrahydropyridine), a toxin selectively affecting dopaminergic neurons [46]. This model simulates the pathological processes known to accompany Parkinson's disease. In the study, rats received unilateral implantation of murine NSCs above the right ventral tegmental area at 1 and 4 weeks following systemic injection of MPTP. Extensive migration of donor cells was seen in both hemispheres of the aged MPTP-treated host brain compared to the young or intact aged brains. Neural transplantation resulted in a gradual reconstruction of the damaged mesostriatal system that was first seen unilaterally followed by bilateral regeneration. On the contrary, no regeneration was seen in MPTP-treated animals that did not receive NSC transplant. When immunohistochemical analysis was done, it showed that the newly formed cells express dopamine, the key neurotransmitter in the striatum. Further analysis showed that even though the restoration of the mesostriatal system was graft-dependent, it was not primarily due to differentiation of the donor NSCs into dopaminergic neurons. While a random and unstructured conversion of NSCs to become mature dopaminergic neurons was seen that contributed to the reconstruction of the mesostrital system, the majority of mesencephalic neurons involved in the recovery process were actually *"rescued" host cells*. These data suggest that the injured host CNS benefited from transplanted NSCs not because the grafted cells replaced the dysfunctional cells, but mainly because the donor cells were able to rescue the damaged neurons. This often ignored new possibility of saving damaged host circuitry and increasing the endogenous regenerative capacity of an adult injured CNS by a plasticity-promoting dialogue between graft and host has now been corroborated in several other studies [21,47-49].

Graft/Host Communication in Head Injury

Communication between grafted and host cells have also been documented to occur in an excitotoxic environment. In an adult rat model of experimentally-induced apoptosis where pyramidal neurons in the neocortex were selectively targeted, NSCs were transplanted into this neurodegenerative environment [50]. Investigators found that 15% of the grafted cells differentiated into pyramidal neurons partially replacing the neuronal population lost due to apoptosis. In addition, it was demonstrated that some 'replacement' neurons were able to form axons that send projections across the corpus callosum to appropriate targets in the contralateral brain hemisphere. These data suggest that even in the presence of a neurodegenerative environment, cues generated by donor and host tissue may be able to direct migration, proliferation, and differentiation of NSCs.

Graft/host communication in injury was also seen during brain development. Using the hypoxic-ischemic injury model, newborn mice were subjected to unilateral carotid ligation combined with reduced ambient oxygen. This model results in extensive hypoxic–ischemic brain (HI) injury throughout the ipsilateral cerebral hemisphere. In this study, the immortalized cells C17.2 were grafted prior to HI injury to a subgroup of animals so that they can integrate into the cytoarchitecture of the host brain during development creating a virtual chimeric brain of host and donor stem cells [51,52] while another subgroup of animals received the C17.2 donor stem cell graft at different intervals following HI injury. The movements and responses of the donor stem cells to HI injury were tracked by evaluating *lacZ* reporter gene expression. The investigators reported that a subpopulation of donor stem cells and host cells transiently re-entered the cell cycle and migrated preferentially to the ischemic site in response to HI injury. Also, it was reported that grafted cells integrated extensively in the injured areas of the brain and even cells transplanted in the intact contralateral hemisphere migrated toward regions of injury. Additionally, a subpopulation of both donor- and host-derived cells differentiated into new neurons and oligodendrocytes, particularly in the penumbral area. Interestingly, a 5-fold increase in donor-derived oligodendrocytes was seen in the injured brain as compared with the intact neocortex. The findings of increased oligodendrocyte production are important because this neural cell type is least likely to regenerate spontaneously following injury to the postnatal CNS. Parallel results were reported in the postnatal spinal cord (SC) injury model using sciatic axotomy resulting in segmental α-motorneuron (MN) degeneration [53]. Following NSC transplantation, a significant portion of the grafted cells migrated toward the injured area and 'repopulated' the ventral horn of the spinal cord. It was reported that approximately 20% of the grafted cells in the ventral horn then differentiated into cells that resemble the lost α-MNs. Again, the importance of these findings must be re-emphasized because α-MNs are normally formed only during fetal development. Taken together, these data suggest the possibility that grafted NSCs whether engineered or not can differentiate, enhance neurite outgrowth and form proper connectivity into the host brain even in a neurodegenerative milieu.

Graft/Host Communication in Genetic Disorders

In verifying that graft/host communication also occurs in CNS disorders with genetic origin, mice with a variety of genetic mutations were tested. These mouse mutants are suitable for conducting well-controlled and well-defined models of complex CNS dysfunctions. For instance, in the *meander tail* (*mea*) mutant, a model characterized by the failure of sufficient granule neurons to develop in certain regions of the cerebellum, NSCs were implanted at birth via the intracerebroventricular method [54]. In this study, the investigators found that the transplanted cells were able to 'repopulate' regions of the cerebellum that lacked sufficient granule neurons. This observation suggests that cells with the potential for multiple fates 'shifted' their mode of differentiation to compensate for a deficiency in a particular cell type. When compared with endogenous NSC differentiation in normal cerebella, most of the donor NSCs in regions deficient in granule neurons pursued a granule neuron phenotype in preference to other neuronal phenotypes suggesting that environmental signals may play a role in 'pushing' undifferentiated, multipotent cells towards replacing the missing cell type.

In a pilot study using another mouse mutant model, active communication between the graft and host cells has also been demonstrated. In the *reeler* (*rl*) mouse, the laminar assignment of neurons in the cortex is profoundly abnormal primarily due to a mutation in the gene encoding the secreted extracellular matrix molecule (ECM), Reelin. In this genetic model, NSC transplantation was done at birth via the intracerebroventricular method with the aim of not only replacing developmentally impaired cells, but also help correct certain aspects of the abnormal brain cytoarchitecture [55]. Investigators reported that the grafted cells were able to replace missing neurons, but more importantly these neurons were found to be in correct laminar position suggesting the possibility that the differentiated NSCs were able to provide molecules (perhaps including Reelin) to guide proper histogenesis. Comparison of the brain cytoarchitecture between the transplanted mutant and wild-type mice showed that the laminar appearance of neurons between these two groups was similar. These findings suggest that CNS disorders characterized by abnormal brain cytoarchitecture may also benefit from stem cell-based therapy.

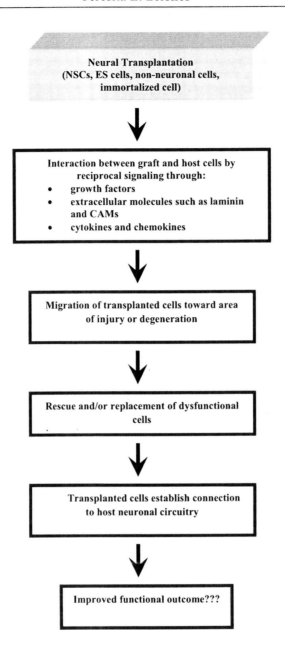

Figure 1. Putative events that occur following neural transplantation. The grafting of NSCs into the damaged CNS initiates a cascade of events starting with the release of signals from donor cells and host tissue to modify their own plasticity-related programs. Depending on the signals released, grafted cells then migrate and repopulate the area of injury where they either: differentiate and replace the dysfunctional neurons or deliver the molecules necessary to enhance the inherent regenerative capacity of the host CNS. The replacement cells then integrate into the cytoarchitecture of the host brain which can lead to functional recovery. The last box have question marks box since the functional significance of graft-induced regeneration and repair is not fully established.

Many CNS diseases, particularly those of genetic origin, are characterized by global degeneration or dysfunction, therefore mutants characterized by CNS-wide white matter disease may provide an ideal model for testing the overall effectiveness of neural cell replacement therapy. The *shiverer* (*shi*) is an appropriate model for widespread CNS white matter disease since the oligodendroglia of this dysmyelinated mouse mutant are dysfunctional because they lack the myelin basic protein gene which is essential for effective myelination [56]. In this mutant model, NSCs were transplanted at birth via the intracerebroventricular technique for diffuse engraftment. Investigators found that a vast majority of donor cells differentiated into oligodendroglia and a subgroup of these glial cells were able to myelinate approximately 40% of host axonal processes. Furthermore, some of the mice demonstrated a decrease in the symptomatic tremor caused by dysmyelination. These results suggest that global CNS pathologies may be amenable to cell replacement. More broadly, findings from these studies have implications for the treatment of neurodevelopmental disorders especially with genetic origins.

The graft-induced "regenerative phenomenon" seen in the above studies is possibly mediated by cellular and molecular mechanisms that modified the brain environment such that intrinsic, albeit latent, regenerative responses by the host were either being triggered, uncovered, or amplified (Fig. 1). It is commonly thought that the observed repair or regeneration seen after NSC transplantation may be attributed solely to the capacity of grafted cells to either deliver the missing neuroactive substances or replace dysfunctional cells. On the other hand, the notion that the host tissue itself may be stimulated by donor-derived cells to release growth promoting molecules so that it can participate in its own repair has been reluctantly acknowledged or otherwise completely ignored; however, based on the results reported in the above studies, this is a thought that should be seriously entertained.

A. Possible Factors That Mediate Graft/Host Communication

The long-range effects of grafted tissue seen in the above studies suggest at least a partial role for secreted and diffusible substances mediating the necessary graft/host interaction (Table 1). Graft/host communications contributing to cell differentiation and the 'regenerative phenomenon' seen in the above studies are likely to include processes similar to those regulating plasticity during development [41]. Such processes include, but are not limited to cell - cell interactions through direct contact or mediated by the extracellular matrix (ECM) and the release of diffusible factors such as Sonic hedgehog [57], tissue specific trophic factors [58], bone morphogenic proteins (BMP) [59], neurotrophins [60,61], and cells of the immune system such as cytokines and chemokines [62,63]. Through intricate intracellular signaling pathways, graft/host communication may lead to the modulation of gene transcription defining the fate of both donor and recipient cells.

A group of molecules that has been well-studied in relation to NSCs is the family of neurotrophic factors which are likely to play a key role in graft-induced host plasticity. Various studies have shown that pools of undifferentiated donor progenitor cells spontaneously express growth factors [53,64-68] such as glial cell line-derived neurotrophic factor (GDNF), neurotrophin-3 (NT-3), brain-derived neurotrophic factor (BDNF), leukemia inhibitory factor (LIF), ciliary neurotrophic factor (CNTF), transforming-growth factor-β (TGF-β) or the newly identified stem cell-derived neural stem/progenitor cell supporting

Table 1. Signaling Molecules Involved in Graft/Host Communications. These molecules are generated by either donor or host cells or both to mediate the multifaceted dialogue that occurs between the grafted cells and host tissue.

Factors Involved in the Dialogue Between Grafted Cells and Host	Functions
Growth factors: • Leukemia inhibitory factor • Ciliary neurotrophic factor • Transforming growth factor-β • Glial cell line-derived neurotrophic factor • Brain-derived neurotrophic factor • Bone morphogenic proteins-2 • Fibroblast growth factor • Stem cell-derived neural stem/progenitor cell supporting factor	- Regulate proliferation and differentiation of transplanted cells
Cell Adhesion Molecules (CAMs): • Integrins • L1 glycoprotein • N-cadherins • N-CAM	- Stabilize connections made by transplanted cells into the host neuronal circuitry - Activate various signaling cascade - Support migration of transplanted cells along the extracellular matrix
Cytokines and Chemokines: • Interleukin-6 • Tumor necrosis factor-α • Macrophage inhibitory protein-3β • CXCR4 – receptor for stromal cell-derived factor-1	- Supports migration of transplanted cells towards dysfunctional areas - Affects proliferation and differentiation of transplanted cells

factor (SDNSF). For example, undifferentiated donor cells and glia adjacent to rescued dopaminergic neurons in MPTP-treated aged mice were found to express GDNF. The protective effects of GDNF were evident not only on dopaminergic neurons in the mesostriatal system but also in the α-MNs located in the ventral horn of the spinal cord. As well, a two-fold increase in the expression of other growth factors such as LIF, CNTF, and TGF-β has been documented in neuronal progenitor cells. FGF is another neurotrophic factor documented to be involved in regulating neural stem cell proliferation both *in vitro* and *in vivo* [69]. Based on these studies, it is believed that growth factors may be necessary in the proliferation and multi-lineage differentiation of both donor and host NSCs.

Another growth-promoting and guidance molecules involved in the plasticity of the developing and grafted CNS are the ECM molecules such as laminin and CAMs. Studies have shown that axonal outgrowth and correct targeting of postsynaptic partners depend critically on the binding of growth cone-associated CAMs to their appropriate receptors because cell motility and migration in the ECM substrates are mediated by adhesion receptors called integrins [70-74]. Once the final axonal links are established, CAMs are found to provide stability to the connections suggesting the ability of these molecules to support cell adhesion and to activate various signaling cascades. CAMs that have been identified to support the migration of transplanted cells along ECMs and their contacts with neuronal, glial, immune, and inflammatory cells are: N-CAM, N-cadherin, and the L1 glycoprotein. L1 glycoprotein is the best-characterized molecule in its class and has been shown to be involved in many events involving plasticity in the developing and adult CNS. Evidence suggests that binding between soluble and neuron-bound forms of L1 glycoprotein is important in cell survival, neurite sprouting, and axonal growth [72]. Mice that overexpress L1 glycoprotein showed that an excess of this molecule can accelerate formation of major motor and sensory fiber tracts and promote the development of these tracts [75]. Overexpression of L1 glycoprotein has also led to the enhanced migration of cerebellar granule cells, patterning of nigral dopaminergic neurons and retinal axons, and possibly enhanced neurogenesis. In humans, mutations in the L1 glycoprotein gene result in a complex disorder in the corpus callosum characterized by agenesis, aphasia, spastic paraplegia and hydrocephalus leading to mental retardation [76]. From these reports it seems reasonable to think that the interactions of cell-bound CAMs with each other and with ECM components can possibly mediate the communication between donor and host cells following neural transplant.

Another often-overlooked group of active molecules that may play a role in mediating graft/host communication are the cytokines and chemokines released after CNS injury and during immune response of the host CNS to neural transplantation. Cytokines have been shown to have a profound effect on the differentiation of NSCs into neurons, astrocytes, and oligodendrocytes [3,77-79]. It is presumed that pro-inflammatory cytokines such as tumor necrosis factor-α (TNF-α) and interleukin-1β (IL-1β) may influence the survival of grafted cells by inducing apoptosis and downregulating the expression of the CAM receptors, integrins, thereby interfering with the ability of donor cells to enhance the regenerative capacity of the host CNS. Conversely, the presence of anti-inflammatory cytokines such as interleukin-1 (IL-6) and IL-10 may promote plasticity in the donor and host cells [80,81]. Confounding the complex role of the immune system in mediating graft/host communication after transplantation is the expression of chemokines. Even though both *in vitro* and *in vivo* studies have demonstrated the dependence of transplanted NSCs on chemokines to migrate from the site of implantation to the region of injury [63,82,83], the role of these immune molecules in neural transplantation is far from being understood. Nevertheless, based on our limited understanding of the role of the immune system on the active dialogue that occurs between the donor cells and host brain following neural transplantation, it can be speculated that the migration, and possibly differentiation of transplanted cells may be influenced by the cytokine and chemokine networks.

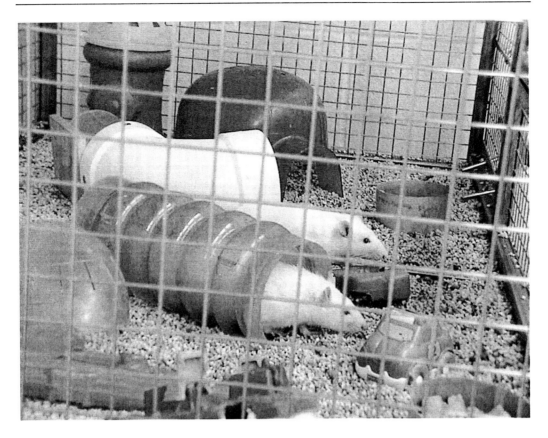

Figure 2. Complex Environment Housing. Rats are usually housed together in a cage filled with a variety of objects. Objects in the home cage are changed at regular intervals to maintain novelty.

B. Enhancing Graft/Host Communication

In some instances, implanted NSCs can easily migrate and engraft in the host brain even if the milieu was degenerative or toxic because of intact cytoarchitecture. Nonetheless, in certain circumstances when there is extensive destruction of the CNS cytoarchitecture, even the use of optimal donor cells has minimal chance of surviving, let alone repairing damaged host cells. In these cases, use of 'scaffolds' may be necessary to optimize the communication between donor and host tissue. Indeed, it has been shown that using a three-dimensional highly porous 'scaffolds' composed of polyglycolic acid (PGA) may act as a bridge between donor and host cells in repairing the damaged CNS circuitry [84-86]. PGA is a synthetic, biodegradable, and highly hydrophobic polymer that has been widely used in clinical medicine. Concerns regarding long-term biocompatibility of PGA should be minimal because PGA looses its mechanical strength in approximately 2-4 weeks after implantation in the body [86]. This length of time is enough to provide an initial matrix to guide cellular organization and growth, allow diffusion of nutrients to the transplanted cells, and become vascularized [84,85]. The efficacy of PGA has been reported in NSC transplant studies involving the brain and spinal cord. At the start, NSCs were co-cultured with PGA *in vitro* for 4 days to allow for the donor cells to adhere to the scaffold and migrate throughout the matrix

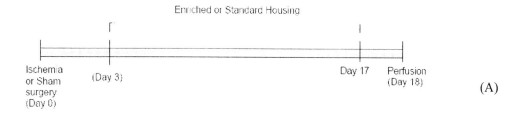

(A)

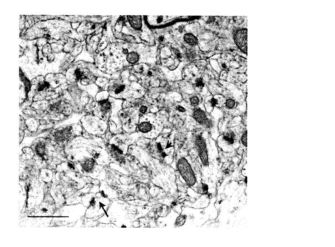

(B)

	Multiple Synaptic Boutons	Perforated PSD
Ischemia EC	3.73 ± 0.39*	2.31 ± 0.38*
Ischemia SC	1.91 ± 0.25	1.38 ± 0.33
Sham EC	4.14 ± 0.42*	2.73 ± 0.42*
Sham SC	1.82 ± 0.44	1.57 ± 0.22

(C)

Figure 3. Enhanced Morphological Plasticity After Cerebral Ischemia May be Mediated by Behavioral Experience (From Briones et al., 2004). (A) Study design. (B) Electron micrograph of the stratum radiatum in the hippocampal area printed at a final magnification of 40,000x illustrating multiple synaptic boutons (long arrow) and perforated synapses (short arrow). Multiple synaptic boutons are synapses formed between an individual axonal bouton and more than one dendritic processes (shafts or spines) while perforated synapses are identified by the presence of a completely partitioned and/or interrupted post-synaptic density. These types of synapse are putatively associated with enhanced efficacy in neurotransmission and a major component of behavioral experience-related plasticity. (C) Number of multiple synaptic boutons and synapses with perforated postsynaptic density per neuron based on stereological analysis. Data are 10^6 synapses per neuron (synaptic density/neuronal density) ± standard error of the mean. *p <0.05. *Abbreviations*: EC – enriched housing, SC – control group, PSD – postsynaptic density. Scale bar = 1 μm.

then the NSC-PGA complex was transplanted in the area of infarction in an experimental HI injury model [84,86]. The investigators reported that the NSC-PGA complex 'repopulated' the area of infarction and became vascularized by the host tissue. Furthermore, with the use of DiI and biotinylated dextrose amine (BDA) as tracers, it was documented that neurite outgrowth of host and donor origins enwrapped the polymer fibers often interconnecting with each other and extended as far as the opposite brain hemisphere. These data suggest that the PGA scaffold may be able to act as an artificial ECM to maximize the reciprocal interaction between the NSC and host tissue.

In a parallel study, NSC seeded on a PGA-based scaffold was transplanted in adult rats with experimentally hemisectioned spinal cord injury [84]. Investigators in this study reported a significant improvement in animal movement following transplantation and at the same time a reduction of necrosis in the surrounding parenchyma was seen, and extensive secondary cell loss, inflammation, and formation of a glial scar were also prevented. Again, using DiI and BDA for tract tracing and GAP-43 (marker for axonal growth) for immunohistochemistry, it was documented that the host tissue displayed regenerated neurites that are not only derived from donor NSCs but also from the recipient spinal cord. These results suggest that the graft/host communication can be augmented to facilitate the repair of damaged neuronal circuitry in the host CNS.

The studies mentioned above provide encouraging evidence that neural tissues can survive transplantation into the adult mammalian brain and spinal cord, integrate and connect with the host nervous system, and influence the host's behavior. Considerable advances have been made over the past decade in understanding the causes of cell death in transplanted tissues, and in developing strategies to improve cell survival, differentiation and long distance axon growth within the host brain. Nevertheless, there are concerns that although grafted cells were able to establish connections with the host brain, the appropriate integration of these connections into the afferent and efferent pathways of the host brain and their contribution to recovery of function have not been fully studied. That is, the functional improvement seen after grafting has not been delineated as different from the spontaneous recovery that occur after CNS injury. It is possible that circuit reconstruction although necessary, might not be sufficient for full functional recovery. There is some validity to this concern since during ontogeny, the growing animal must not only develop the right anatomical structures and systems, but also acquire and refine appropriate patterns of behavior through learning and experience [87]. The influence of experience and physical activity on CNS plasticity has each been extensively investigated in its own right. Data from animals and humans suggest that appropriate rehabilitation through experience, practice, and retraining is necessary to aid spontaneous recovery and reacquire lost function after CNS injury [88-93]. But the degree to which these rehabilitation strategies can enhance the active communication between graft and host cells is not clear. Although limited, experimental evidence suggests that rehabilitation training may be important in enhancing the plasticity of, and functional recovery provided by neural grafts (Table 2).

The mechanisms by which behavioral experience can influence brain structure and function first received attention after Hebb's observations and theoretical proposals that learning is represented in the brain by synaptic changes in response to repeated concurrent activation [94]. These fundamental concepts were subsequently confirmed at the cellular and molecular levels in various organisms ranging from simple to complex [95]. The inherent regenerative capacity of the adult brain to respond to injury may also be influenced by behavioral experience [90]. Our group has demonstrated that enriched housing condition (Fig. 2) following global cerebral ischemia enhanced the spontaneous recovery from injury evidenced by the alteration in synaptic morphology at the site of infarction (Fig. 3). Thus, it is possible that the intrinsic plasticity of the adult CNS to recover from injury may be augmented by behavioral experience. Consequently, the possibility exists that rehabilitation strategies following neural transplantation may enhance the functional integration of neural grafts into the host neuronal circuitry leading to complete behavioral recovery.

Table 2. EC Studies on Rehabilitation Effects on Graft Survival and Function.

Injury Model	Graft Source	Rehabilitation Strategy	Morphological Results	Functional Results	References
Fimbria-fornix aspiration lesion	Fetal septal tissue	Environmental enrichment	Increased neurite outgrowth in the hippocampus	Improved performance in the Hebb-Williams maze	100
Focal ischemia (MCAO)	Fetal neocortical tissue	Environmental enrichment	No effect on size of infarction but decreased thalamic atrophy was seen	Improved posture and performance in traversing the rotating pole	99 and 101
Lesion of the nigrostriatal dopamine pathway	Fetal striatal tissue	Enriched environment	Increased graft survival and formation of dopaminergic neurons	Improved performance in the delayed alternation and rotation tasks	19, 96 and 98
Cortical aspiration	Fetal cortex	Environmental enrichment	No effects on lesion size	Improved performance in the beam walking task	97
Lesion of the striatum	Fetal striatal tissue	Environmental enrichment	Enriched housing condition increased the development of striatal-like neurons	Improved performance in the staircase walking task	102

The literature on the behavioral effects of rehabilitation training following cell-based therapy is very limited. Some studies have shown that grafts that are rich in cholinergic neurons derived from the embryonic basal forebrain were able to reverse various cognitive impairments associated with cholinergic depletion in the rat cortex and hippocampus caused by ageing or experimental lesions [19,96-102]. In particular, grafted cells in the dorsal neocortex resulted in increased cholinergic fiber outgrowth that was greater in rats that were housed in an enriched or complex environment (EC) as compared to rats kept in standard laboratory cages. The difference in cholinergic fiber outgrowth seen in these studies was particularly marked at 4 weeks after grafting, but seemed to decrease by 10 weeks, suggesting that the greatest effect of complex environment housing might be during the initial interactions between the graft and host cells. Interestingly, the reports on behavioral recovery following EC housing and neural transplantation are conflicting where others demonstrated amelioration in functional deficits while others have shown no improvement in behavior. These conflicting results may be a function of differences in behavioral tests used, length of time in EC, and timing of grafts after injury. The behavioral test used ranged from the simple task of motor asymmetry, such as rotation, postural position and balance on a rotating rod to the more complex test of skilled forelimb reaching task and maze learning. Additionally, the length of EC housing used in these studies ranged from 2 to 10 months while timing of grafts range from immediately after to several days after lesion. Timing of graft after injury may be the most important variable because it is possible that delaying the lesion - graft interval may reduce the opportunities for the grafts to establish the necessary afferent and efferent innervations to become fully functional. From these studies, it is clear that the role of rehabilitation training in mediating the successful communication between the grafted cells and host tissue deserves additional investigation. Since neuronal reorganization that occurs after CNS injury have been compared to the plasticity observed in development, involving sprouting and pruning stages, each under behavioral experience-dependent control [87], it is possible that a similar mechanism may be necessary for the 'appropriate' integration of grafted cell into the host circuitry.

Conclusions

In this review, the multifaceted dialogue that occurs between the graft and host tissue, and the graft evoked host plasticity has been highlighted as central in understanding the role of neurotransplantation in restorative medicine. The various mechanisms that may mediate the active communication between the graft and host tissue have also been discussed although the role of some molecules (e.g. cytokines and chemokines) are less understood than others (e.g. growth factors and CAMs). Despite our continuing efforts to gain insight on the interactions between graft and host tissue, NSC transplantation after CNS injury is still fraught with problems such as inconsistent and poor cell survival, and limited differentiation of donor cells to neuronal versus glial phenotypes. To face these challenges, further studies need to be done on the changes that occur in the CNS environment during various types of injuries as well as the factors in the environment that might interfere with NSC survival and differentiation. Also, since it is commonly acknowledged that the CNS environment after injury may not be accommodating to neural grafting, more attention is needed on how to shift the balance between permissive and non-permissive milieu to favor successful transplantation. Lastly, consideration must be given to the fact that replacing lost cells and reconstructing damaged circuits of the brain although necessary, may not be sufficient for recovery of function after injury. Thus, the possibility that neural transplantation and rehabilitation training may have complementary roles in promoting full functional recovery deserves further attention.

References

1.   Gage FH, Kempermann G, Palmer TD, Peterson DA, Ray J: Multipotent progenitor cells in the adult dentate gyrus. *Journal of Neurobiology* 1998, 36:249-266.
2.   Altman J, Das GD: Autoradiographic examination of the effects of enriched environment on the rate of glial multiplication in the adult rat brain. *Nature* 1964, 204:1161-1163.

3. Xiao BG, Link H: Immune regulation within the central nervous system. *Journal of Neurological Science* 1998, 157:1-12.

4. Levison SW, Goldman JE: Multipotential and lineage restricted precursors coexist in the mammalian perinatal subventicular zone. *Journal of Neuroscience Research* 1997, 48:83-94.

5. Mayer-Proschel M, Kalyani AJ, Mujtaba T, Rao MS: Isolation of lineage-restricted neuronal precursors from multipotent neuroepithelial stem cells. *Neuron* 1997, 19:773-785.

6. Clarke DL, Johansson CB, Wilbertz J, Veress B, Nilsson E, Karlstrom H, Lendahl U, Frisen J: Generalized Potential of Adult Neural Stem Cells. *Science* 2000, 288:1660-1663.

7. Meyerrose TE, Herrbrich P, Hess DA, Nolta JA: Immune-deficient mouse models for analysis of human stem cells. *Biotechniques* 2003, 35:1262-1272.

8. Ourednik V, Ourednik J, Flax JD, Zawada WM, Hutt C, Yang C, Park KI, Kim SU, Sidman RL, Freed CR, et al.: Segregation of human neural stem cells in the developing primate forebrain. *Science* 2001, 293:1820-1824.

9. Lois C, Alvarez-Buylla A: Proliferating subventricular zone cells in the adult mammalian forebrain can differentiate into neurons and glia. *Proceedings National Academy of Science* 1993, 90:2074-2077.

10. Johansson CB, Momma S, Clarke DL, Risling M, Lendahl U, Frisen J: Identification of neural stem cell in the adult mammalian central nervous system. *Cell* 1999, 96:25-34.

11. Carlen M, Cassidy RM, Brismar H, Smith GA, Enquist LW, Frisen J: Functional Integration of Adult-Born Neurons. *Current Biology* 2002, 12:606-608.

12. Palmer TD, Schwartz PH, Taupin P, Kaspar B, Stein SA, Gage FH: Cell culture: progenitor cells from human brain after death. *Nature* 2001, 411:42-43.

13. Labat ML: Stem cells and the promise of eternal youth: embryonic versus adult stem cells. *Biomedecine & Pharmacotherapy* 2001, 55:179-185.

14. Flax JD, Aurora S, Yang C: Engraftable human neural stem cells respond to developmental cues, replace neurons, and express foreign genes. *Nature Biotechnology* 1998, 16:1033-1039.

15. Bain G, Kitchens D, Yao M, Huettner JE, Gootlieb DI: Embryonic stem cells express neuronal properties in vitro. *Developmental Biology* 1995, 168:342-357.

16. Liu S, Qu Y, Stewart TJ, Howard MJ, Chakrabortty S, Holekamp TF, McDonald JW: Embryonic stem cells differentiate into oligodendrocytes and myelinate in culture and after spinal cord transplantation. *Proceedings National Academy of Science* 2000, 97:6126-6131.

17. Brustle O, Jones KN, Learish RD, Karram K, Choudhary K, Wiestler OD, Duncan ID, McKay RD: Embryonic stem cell-derived glial precursors: a source of myelinating transplants. *Science* 1999, 285:754-756.

18. Sorensen JC, Grabowski M, Zimmer J, Johansson BB: Fetal neocortical tissue blocks implanted in brain infarction of adult rats interconnect with the host brain. *Experimental Neurology* 1996, 138:227-235.

19. Döbrössy MD, Dunnett SB: Motor training effects on recovery of function after striatal lesions and striatal grafts. *Experimental Neurology* 2003, 184:274-284.

20. Chu K, Kim M, Park K-I, Jeong S-W, Park H-K, Jung K-H, Lee S-T, Kang L, Lee K, Park D-K: Human neural stem cells improve sensorimotor deficits in the adult rat brain with experimental focal ischemia. *Brain Research* 2004, 1016:145-153.

21. Englund U, Bjorklund A, Wictorin K, Lindvall O, Kokaia M: Grafted neural stem cells develop into functional pyramidal neurons and integrate into host cortical circuitry. *Proceedings National Academy of Science* 2002, 99:17089-17094.

22. Wernig M, Benninger F, Schmandt T, Rade M, Tucker KL, Bussow H, Beck H, Brustle O: Functional Integration of embryonic stem cell-derived neurons in vivo. *Journal of Neuroscience* 2004, 24:5258-5268.

23. Freed CR, Greene PE, Breeze RE, Tsai W-Y, DuMouchel W, Kao R, Dillon S, Winfield H, Culver S, Trojanowski JQ, et al.: Transplantation of embryonic dopamine neurons for severe Parkinson's disease. *New England Journal of Medicine* 2001, 344:710-719.

24. Kirik D, Björklund A: Histological analysis of fetal dopamine cell suspension grafts in two patients with Parkinson's disease gives promising results. *Brain* 2005, 128:1478-1479.

25. Englund U, Fricker-Gates RA, Lundberg C, Björklund A, Wictorin K: Transplantation of human neural progenitor cells into the neonatal rat brain: extensive migration and differentiation with long-distance axonal projections. *Experimental Neurology* 2002, 173:1-21.

26. Eriksson C, Björklund A, Wictorin K: Neuronal differentiation following transplantation of expanded mouse neurosphere cultures derived from different embryonic forebrain regions. *Experimental Neurology* 2003, 184:615-635.

27. Jensen JB, Björklund A, Parmar M: Striatal neuron differentiation from neurosphere-expanded progenitors depends on Gsh2 expression. *Journal of Neuroscience* 2004, 24:6958-6967.

28. Tabar V, Panagiotakos G, Greenberg ED, Chan BK, Sadelain M, Gutin PH, Studer L: Migration and differentiation of neural precursors derived from human embryonic stem cells in the rat brain. *Nature Biotechnology* 2005, 23:601-606.

29. Studer L, Tabar V, McKay R: Transplantation of expanded mesencephalic precursors leads to recovery in parkinsonian rats. *Nature Neuroscience* 1998, 1:290-295.

30. Björklund A, Lindvall O: Cell replacment therapies for central nervous system disorders. *Nature Neuroscience* 2000, 3:537-544.

31. Veizovic T, Beech JS, Stroemer RP, Watson WP, Hodges H: Resolution of stroke deficits following contralateral grafts of conditionally immortal neuroepithelial stem cells. *Stroke* 2001, 32:1012-1019.

32. Terada N, Hamazaki T, Oka M, Hoki M, Mastalerz DM, Nakano Y, Meyer EM, Morel L, Petersen BE, Scott EW: Bone marrow cells adopt the phenotype of other cells by spontaneous cell fusion. *Nature* 2002, 416:542-545.

33. Kleppner SR, Robinson KA, Trojanowski JQ, Lee VM: Transplanted human neurons derived from a teratocarcinoma cell line mature, integrate, and survive for

over 1 year in the nude mouse brain. *Journal of Comparative Neurology* 1995, 357:618-632.

34. Borlongan CV, Tajima Y, Trojanowski JQ, Lee VM, Sanberg PR: Transplantation of cryopreserved human embryonal carcinoma-derived neurons (NT2N cells) promotes functional recovery in ischemic rats. *Experimental Neurology* 1998, 149:310-321.

35. Kondziolka D, Wechsler L, Goldstein S, Meltzer C, Thulbon KR, Gebel J, Jannetta PJ, DeCesare S, Elder EM, McGrogan M, et al.: Transplantation of cultured human neuronal cells for patients with stroke. *Neurology* 2000, 55:565-569.

36. Saporta S, Makoui AS, Willing AE, Daadi M, Cahill DW, Sanberg PR: Functional recovery after complete contusion injury to the spinal cord and transplantation of human neuroteratocarcinoma neurons in rats. *Journal of Neurosurgery* 2002, 97:63-68.

37. Snyder EY, Deitcher DL, Walsh CA, Arnold-Aldea S, Hartwieg EA, Cepko CL: Multipotent neural cell lines can engraft and participate in development of mouse cerebellum. *Cell* 1992, 68:33-51.

38. Park K: Transplantation of neural stem cells: cellular and gene therapy for hypoxic-ischemic brain injury. *Yonsei Medical Journal* 2000, 41:825-835.

39. Franklin RJM, Bayley SA, Blakemore WF: Transplanted CG4 Cells (an oligodendrocyte progenitor cell line) survive, migrate, and contribute to repair of areas of demyelination in X-Irradiated and damaged spinal cord but not in normal spinal cord. *Experimental Neurology* 1996, 137:263-276.

40. Tourbah A, Linnington C, Bachelin C, Avellana-Adalid V, Wekerle H, A. Baron-Van Evercooren: Inflammation promotes survival and migration of the CG4 oligodendrocyte progenitors transplanted in the spinal cord of both inflammatory and demyelinated EAE rats. *Journal of Neuroscience Research* 1997, 50:853-861.

41. Ourednik J, Ourednik W, Loos Vd: Do foetal neural grafts induce repair by the injured juvenile neocortex? *Neuroreport* 1993, 5:133-136.

42. Andres FL, Van der Loos H: Removal and re-implantation of the parietal cortex of the neonatal mouse: consequences for the barrel field. *Brain Reseach* 1985, 352:115-121.

43. Ourednik J, Ourednik W, Mitchell DE: Remodeling of lesioned kitten visual cortex after xenotransplantation of fetal mouse neopallidium. *Journal of Comparative Neurology* 1998, 395:91-111.

44. Ourednik V, Ourednik J: Graft/host relationships in the developing and regenerating CNS of mammals. *Annals New York Academy of Science* 2005, 1049:172-184.

45. Valoušková V, Gálik J: Unilateral grafting of fetal neocortex into a cortical cavity improves healing of a symmetric lesion in the contralateral cortex of adult rats. *Neuroscience Letters* 1995, 186:103-106.

46. Ourednik J, Ourednik V, Lynch WP, Schachner M, Snyder EY: Neural stem cells display an inherent mechanism for rescuing dysfunctional neurons. *Nature Biotechnology* 2002, 20:1103-1110.

47. Fujiwara Y, Tanaka N, Ishida O, Fujimoto Y, Murakami T, Kajihara H, Yasunaga Y, Ochi M: Intravenously injected neural progenitor cells of transgenic rats can migrate to the injured spinal cord and differentiate into neurons, astrocytes and oligodendrocytes. *Neuroscience Letters* 2004, 366:287-291.

48. McDonald JW, Becker D, Holekamp TF, Howard M, Liu S, Lu A, Lu J, Platik MM, Qu Y, Stewart T, et al.: Repair of the injured spinal cord and the potential of embryonic stem cell transplantation. *Journal of Neurotrauma* 2004, 21:383-393.

49. Pfeifer K, Vroemen M, Blesch A, Weidner N: Adult neural progenitor cells provide a permissive guiding substrate for corticospinal axon growth following spinal cord injury. *European Journal of Neuroscience* 2004, 20:1695-1704.

50. Snyder EY, Yoon C, Flax JD, Macklis JD: Multipotent neural precursors can differentiate toward replacement of neurons undergoing targeted apoptotic degeneration in adult mouse neocortex. *Proceedings National Academy of Science* 1997, 94:663-668.

51. Park KI, Liu S, Flax JD, Nissim S, Stieg PE, Synder EY: Transplantation of neuronal progenitor and stem-like cells: development insights may suggest new therapies for spinal cord and other CNS dysfunction. *Journal of Neurotrauma* 1999, 16:675-687.

52. Liu Y, Himes BT, Solowska J, Moul J, Chow SY, Park KI, Tessler A, Murray M, Snyder EY, Fischer I: Intraspinal Delivery of Neurotrophin-3 Using Neural Stem Cells Genetically Modified by Recombinant Retrovirus. *Experimental Neurology* 1999, 158:9-26.

53. Himes BT, Liu Y, Solowska JM, Snyder EY, Fischer I, Tessler A: Transplants of cells genetically modified to express neurotrophin-3 rescue axotomized Clarke's nucleus neurons after spinal cord hemisection in adult rats. *Journal of Neuroscience Research* 2001, 65:549-564.

54. Rosario C, Yandava B, Kosaras B, Zurakowski D, Sidman R, Snyder E: Differentiation of engrafted multipotent neural progenitors towards replacement of missing granule neurons in meander tail cerebellum may help determine the locus of mutant gene action. *Development* 1997, 124:4213-4224.

55. Park KI, Ourednik J, Ourednik V, Taylor RM, Aboody KS, Auguste KI, Lachyankar MB: Global gene and cell replacement strategies via stem cells. *Gene Therapy* 2002, 9:613-624.

56. Yandava BD, Billinghurst L, Synder EY: "Global"cell replacement is feasible via neural stem cell transplantation: evidence from the dysmyelinated shrverer mouse brain. *Proceedings National Academy of Science* 1999, 96:7029-7034.

57. Rowitch DH, St.-Jacques B, Lee SMK, Flax JD, Snyder EY, McMahon AP: Sonic hedgehog Regulates Proliferation and Inhibits Differentiation of CNS Precursor Cells. *Journal of Neuroscience* 1999, 19:8954-8965.

58. Lu P, Jones LL, Snyder EY, Tuszynski MH: Neural stem cells constitutively secrete neurotrophic factors and promote extensive host axonal growth after spinal cord injury. *Experimental Neurology* 2003, 181:115-129.

59. Kleber M, Lee H-Y, Wurdak H, Buchstaller J, Riccomagno MM, Ittner LM, Suter U, Epstein DJ, Sommer L: Neural crest stem cell maintenance by combinatorial Wnt and BMP signaling. *Journal of Cell Biology* 2005, 169:309-320.

60. Sommer L, Rao MS: Neural stem cells and regulation of cell number. *Progress in Neurobiology* 2002, 66:1-8.

61. Philips MF, Mattiasson G, Wieloch T, Björklund A, Johansson BB, Tomasevic G, Matinez-Serrano A, Lenzlinger PM, Sinson G, Grady MS, et al.: Neuroprotective and behavioral efficacy of nerve growth factor-transfected hippocampal progenitor cell transplants after experimental brain injury. *Journal of Neurosurgery* 2001, 94:765-774.

62. Wuu YD, Pampfer S, CVanderheyden I, Lee KH, De Hertogh R: Impact of tumor necrosis factor alpha on mouse embryonic stem cells. *Biology of Reproduction* 1998, 58:1416-1424.

63. Rezaie P, Trillo-Pazos G, Everall IP, Male DK: Expression of beta-chemokines and chemokine receptors in human fetal astrocyte and microglial co-cultures: potential role of chemokines in the developing CNS. *Glia* 2002, 37:64-75.

64. Ahn Y-H, Bensadoun J-C, Aebischer P, Zurn AD, Seiger A, Bjorklund A, Lindvall O, Wahlberg L, Brundin P, Kaminski Schierle GS: Increased fiber outgrowth from xeno-transplanted human embryonic dopaminergic neurons with co-implants of polymer-encapsulated genetically modified cells releasing glial cell line-derived neurotrophic factor. *Brain Research Bulletin* 2005, 66:135-142.

65. Rolletschek A, Chang H, Guan K, Czyz J, Meyer M, Wobus AM: Differentiation of embryonic stem cell-derived dopaminergic neurons is enhanced by survival-promoting factors. *Mechanisms of Development* 2001, 105:93-104.

66. Toda H, Tsuji M, Nakano I, Kobuke K, Hayashi T, Kasahara H, Takahashi J, Mizoguchi A, Houtani T, Sugimoto T, et al.: Stem cell-derived neural stem/progenitor cell supporting factor is an autocrine/paracrine survival factor for adult neural stem/progenitor cells. *Journal of Biological Chemistry* 2003, 278:35491-35500.

67. Galli R, Pagano SF, Gritti A, Vescovi AL: Regulation of neuronal differentiation in human CNS stem cell progeny by leukemia inhibitory factor. *Developmental Neuroscience* 2000, 22:86-95.

68. Manabe Y, Nagano I, Gazi MS, Murakami T, Shiote M, Shoji M, Kitagawa H, Abe K: Glial cell line-derived neurotrophic factor protein prevents motor neuron loss of transgenic mice model for amyotrophic lateral sclerosis. *Neurological Research* 2003, 25:195-200.

69. Kinkl N, Hageman GS, Sahel JA, Hicks D: Fibroblast growth factor receptor (FGFR) and candidate signaling molecule distribution within rat and human retina. *Molecular Vision* 2002, 8:149-160.

70. Cremer H, Chazal G, Goridis C, Represa A: NCAM is essential for axonal growth and fasciculation in the hippocampus. *Molecular and Cellular Neuroscience* 1997, 8:323-335.

71. Dihne M, Bernreuther C, Sibbe M, Paulus W, Schachner M: A new role for the cell adhesion molecule L1 in neural precursor cell proliferation, differentiation, and

transmitter-specific subtype generation. *Journal of Neuroscience* 2003, 23:6638-6650.

72. Ourednik J, Ourednik V, Bastmeyer M, Schachner M: Ectopic expression of the neural cell adhesion molecule L1 in astrocytes leads to changes in the development of the corticospinal tract. *European Journal of Neuroscience* 2001, 14:1464-1476.

73. Brummendorf T, Kenwrick S, Rathjen FG: Neural cell recognition molecule L1: from cell biology to human hereditary brain malformations. *Current Opinion in Neurobiology* 1998, 8:87-97.

74. Huang EJ, Reichardt LF: Neurotrophins: roles in neuronal development and function. *Annual Review in Neuroscience* 2001, 24:677-736.

75. Ourednik V, Schachner M, Snyder EY, Lynch WP, Ourednik J: Rescue of impaired host dopaminergic neurons and the role of overexpressed neural cell adhesion molecule L1 in aged mice grafted with neural stem cells (NSCs). *Experimental Neurology* 2003, 181:101.

76. Kamiguchi H, Hlavin ML, Yamasaki M, Lemmon V: Adhesion molecules and inherited diseases of the human nervous system. *Annual Review in Neuroscience* 1998, 21:97-125.

77. Imitola J, Comabella M, Chandraker AK, Dangond F, Sayegh MH, Synder EY, Khoury SJ: Neural stem/progenitor cells express co-stimulatory molecules that are differentially upregulated by inflammatory and apoptotic stimuli. *American Journal of Pathology* 2004, 164:1615-1625.

78. Cammer W: Effects of TNF-alpha on immature and mature oligodendrocytes and their progenitors in vitro. *Brain Reseach* 2000, 864:213-219.

79. Shohami E, Ginis I, Hallenbeck JM: Dual role of tumor necrosis factor alpha in brain injury. *Cytokine Growth Factor Reviews* 1999, 10:119-130.

80. Qin L, Chavin KD, Ding Y, Tahara H, Favaro JP, Woodward JE, Suzuki T, Robbins PD, Lotze MT, Bromberg JS: Retro-virus mediated gene transfer of viral IL-10 gene prolongs murine cardiac allograft survival. *Journal of Immunology* 1996, 156:2316-2323.

81. Penkowa M, Giralt M, Lago N, Camats J, Carrasco J, Hernandez J, Molinero A, Campbell IL, Hidalgo J: Astrocyte-targeted expression of IL-6 protects the CNSagainst a focal brain injury. *Experimental Neurology* 2003, 181:130-148.

82. Tran PB, Miller RJ: Chemokine receptors in the brain: a developing story. *Journal of Comparative Neurology* 2003, 457:1-6.

83. Imitola J, Raddassi K, Park KI, Mueller F-J, Nieto M, Teng YD, Frenkel D, Li J, Sidman RL, Walsh CA, et al.: Directed migration of neural stem cells to sites of CNS injury by the stromal cell-derived factor 1-α/CXC chemokine receptor 4 pathway. *Proceedings National Academy of Science* 2004, 101:18117-18122.

84. Teng YD, Lavik EB, Qu X, Park KI, Ourednik J, Zurakowski D, Langer R, Snyder EY: Functional recovery following traumatic spinal cord injury mediated by a unique polymer scaffold seeded with neural stem cells. *Proceedings National Academy of Science* 2002, 99:3024-3029.

85. Bakshi A, Fisher O, Dagci T, Himes BT, Fischer I, Lowman A: Mechanically engineered hydrogel scaffolds for axonal growth and angiogenesis after transplantation in spinal cord injury. *J Neurosurgery of Spine* 2004, 1:322-329.

86. Park KI, Teng YD, Snyder EY: The injured brain interacts reciprocally with neural stem cells supported by scaffolds to reconstitute lost tissue. *Nature Biotechnology* 2002, 20:1111-1117.

87. Xerri C, Coq JO, Merzenich MM, Jenkins WM: Experience-induced plasticity of cutaneous maps in the primary somatosensory cortex of adult monkey and rats. *Journal of Physiology (Paris)* 1996, 90:277-287.

88. Robertson IH, Murre JMJ: Rehabilitation of brain damage: brain plasticity and principles of guided recovery. *Psychological Bulletin* 1999, 125:544-575.

89. Jones TA, Chu CJ, Grande LA, Gregory AD: Motor skills training enhances lesion-induced structural plasticity in the motor cortex of adult rats. *The Journal of Neuroscience* 1999, 19:10153-10163.

90. Briones TL, Suh E, Jozsa L, Hattar H, Chai J, Wadowska M: Behaviorally-induced ultrastructural plasticity in the hippocampal region after cerebral ischemia. *Brain Research* 2004, 997:137-146.

91. Luke LM, Allred RP, Jones TA: Unilateral ischemic sensorimotor cortical damage induces contralesional synaptogenesis and enhances skilled reaching with the ipsilateral forelimb in adult male rats. *Synapse* 2004, 54:187-199.

92. Briones TL, Therrien B, Metzger B: Effects of environment on enhancing functional plasticity following cerebral ischemia. *Biological Research for Nursing* 2000, 1:299-309.

93. Young D, Lawlor PA, Leone P, Gragunow M, During MJ: Environmental enrichment inhibits spontaneous apoptosis, prevents seizures and is neuroprotective. *Nature Medicine* 1999, 5:448-453.

94. Hebb DO: *The Organization of Behavior*. New York: Wiley; 1949.

95. van Praag H, Kempermann G, Gage FH: Neural consequences of environmental enrichment. *Nature Reviews Neuroscience* 2000, 1:191-198.

96. Döbrössy MD, Le Moal M, Montaron M-F, Abrous N: Influence of environment on the efficacy of intrastriatal dopaminergic grafts. *Experimental Neurology* 2000, 165:172-183.

97. Christie MA, Dalrymple-Alford JC: Behavioural consequences of frontal cortex grafts and enriched environments after sensorimotor cortex lesions. *Journal of Neural Transplantation and Plasticity* 1995, 5:199-210.

98. Döbrössy MD, Dunnett SB: Environmental enrichment affects striatal graft morphology and functional recovery. *European Journal of Neuroscience* 2004, 19:159-168.

99. Grabowski M, Sorensen JC, Mattsson B, Zimmer J, Johansson BB: Influence of an enriched environment and cortical grafting on functional outcome in brain infarcts of adult rats. *Experimental Neurology* 1995, 133:96-102.

100. Kelche C, Dalrymple-Alford JC, Will B: Housing condition modulate the effects of intracerebral grafts in rats with brain lesions. *Behavioral Brain Research* 1988, 28:287-295.

101. Mattsson B, Sorensen JC, Zimmer J, Johansson BB: Neural grafting to experimental neocortical infarcts improves behavioral outcome and reduces thalamic atrophy in rats housed in enriched but not in standard environments. *Stroke* 1997, 28:1225-1231.

102. Döbrössy MD, Dunnett SB: Training specificity, graft development and graft-mediated functional recovery in a rodent model of Huntington's disease. *Neuroscience* 2005, 132:543-552.

In: Neural Stem Cell Research
Editor: Eric V. Grier, pp. 27-50

ISBN: 1-59454-846-3
© 2006 Nova Science Publishers, Inc.

Chapter 2

ROLES OF EXTRACELLULAR MATRIX MOLECULES IN NEURAL STEM CELL DEVELOPMENT AND THE EXAMPLE OF TENASCIN-C

*Jeremy Garwood**

Laboratoire de Neurobiologie du Développement et de la Régénération,
CNRS Centre de Neurochimie, 67084 Strasbourg, France

Abstract

In situ, neural stem cells are located in a niche that consists of a restricted set of cell types and contains a specialised microenvironment composed of soluble factors, membrane-bound molecules and extracellular matrix components. The roles of extracellular matrix (ECM) molecules in the development, maintenance and plasticity of the central nervous system have been the subject of increasing study. The in vivo expression profile of these molecules, notably in and leading out of the germinal zones, especially the subventricular zone, has given clues as to their influence on a range of developmental processes, including proliferation, migration, survival, and process outgrowth. In vitro studies on primary cell cultures and neural stem cell-derived neurospheres have confirmed cell-type specific effects of ECM molecules such as the glycoprotein, Tenascin-C, the proteoglycan, phosphacan, and of post-translational carbohydrate modifications on ECM and cell adhesion molecules, such as PSA, Lewis-X and HNK-1. Recent data derived from analysis of transgenic knockout mice is further contributing to an understanding of the roles of these ECM molecules in CNS development and regeneration. Most notably, Tenascin-C has now been shown to alter the responsiveness of neural stem cells and stem-cell derived precursors to several growth factors, including bFGF, BMP-4, and PDGF, thereby affecting the generation of a stem cell niche within the subventricular zone by acting to orchestrate growth factor signalling and the rate of neural stem cell development. The nature of these effects on neural stem cells and oligodendrocyte precursor cell behaviour is considered in more detail.

---

* Email: garwood@neurochem.u-strasbg.fr

Introduction

Genetic Versus Environmental Factors

The differentiation and morphogenesis of animal tissue involves a diversity of interactions between cells and their environment. Most cells in multicellular organisms are in contact with an intricate meshwork of interacting extracellular collagens, proteoglycans and adhesion proteins, as well as growth factors, chemokines and cytokines. Together, these components constitute the extracellular matrix (ECM) and many potentially important interactions occur between cells and the extracellular matrix (ECM) surrounding them (Gumbiner, 1996; Streuli, 1999; Garwood *et al.*, 2002; Kleinman *et al.*, 2003)(Figure 1).

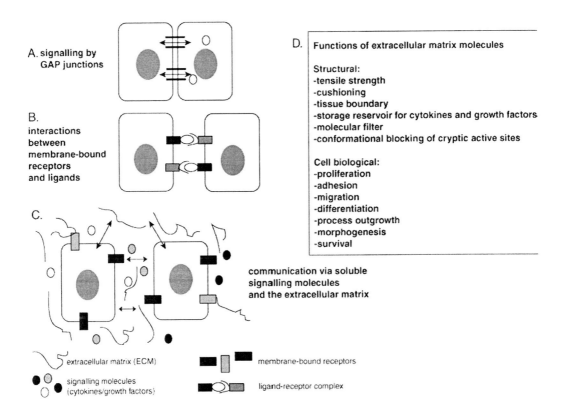

Figure 1. Simplified Overview Of Basic Mechanisms Of Cell-Cell Communication And The Presence Of The Extracellular Matrix.
A.   GAP junctions permit a direct exchange between cells
B.   Close cell-cell contact can result in the formation of trans-signalling complexes between cell membrane-bound receptors and ligands on adjacent cells
C.   Communication through the extracellular space may imply a range of soluble signalling molecules, such as growth factors, chemokines and cytokines, as well as molecules of the extracellular matrix. These may interact with each other as well as with receptors on the cell membrane, and be influenced by changes in the local microenvironment, such as pH and the concentration of ions.
The box presents a summary of the principle structural and biological roles that extracellular molecules have been shown to play in mammals.

In general, a distinction has been made in the development of the organism between events which are genetically determined (intrinsic) and those which are more subject to localised environmental factors (extrinsic). The intrinsic factors apparently underlie the earliest stages of embryogenesis, early stages of proliferation and stem cell determination and the initial migration out of the germinal zones of proliferation, while the more developed the tissue becomes, especially in the adult, and the further the cells pass along the route of morphogenetic development, the greater is the role of the extrinsic environmental cues in determining the cell's "behaviour". Developing cells are embedded in complex fields of mechanical tension and diffusible biochemical signals. This constantly changing pattern of spatial and temporal information for each cell is largely generated by the cells themselves, and represents the major environmental forces that drive the sequence of developmental processes. The dynamic interactions between these environmental influences and the cells' response to them account for the considerable transformations which the cells undergo during periods of growth and survival, migration and sorting, and morphological and biochemical differentiation. There is increasing evidence however, that ECM components can play crucial roles in cellular microenvironments or niches even at very early developmental stages. For example, the laminin γ1 chain, synthesized at the two-cell stage, appears to be the first ECM molecule expressed, and serves as an initial matrix scaffolding. Mice that lack the gene encoding laminin γ1 fail to organize a basement membrane matrix and die at embryonic day 5.5 and stem cells that lack this gene cannot form an epiblast (Gustafsson & Fassler, 2000; Li *et al.*, 2002).

The key characteristics of stem cells are self-renewal and multipotency with the capacity to generate cell precursors that can migrate and differentiate into determined mature cell types. In vivo, these cells are contacted by various soluble and insoluble ECM components that influence their differentiation (Czyz & Wobus, 2001).

The large number of ECM molecules and their interactions with each other define unique biological matrices important in morphogenesis (Kleinman *et al.*, 2003). There is considerable variation in the amount and type of specific components present in ECMs in different tissues and at different stages of development (Streuli, 1999). In order to reflect the realisation of the existence of such environmental complexity within animal tissue, the concept of cellular niche has been derived from the domain of ecology (Spradling *et al.*, 2001). The existence of a particular cellular niche with unique properties regulating their self-renewal, activation, differentiation and migration has in particular been postulated in the case of multipotential stem and precursor cells in developed and adult tissue. These progenitor cells tend to lie embedded as discrete sub-populations within restricted regions of mature tissue. Common components of stem cell niches are signalling from somatic cells, a basement membrane for cell anchoring, and extracellular matrices (ECMs), which modulate the adhesiveness and activity of signalling molecules (Czyz & Wobus, 2001; Doetsch, 2003).

Extracellular Matrix: Composition and Roles of ECM Molecules In Tissue

The ECM in neural tissues is a complex and dynamic entity composed of many types of molecules that have distinct patterns of spatial and temporal expression. Many ECM components, originally discovered in non-neural tissues, are also present in developing neural tissues, including fibronectin, laminin, vitronectin, collagens, proteoglycans, and thrombospondin (Pearlman & Sheppard, 1996; Julliard & Hartmann, 1998; Garwood et al., 2002).

The extracellular space is filled with an assortment of molecules, ranging from small ionic species to huge polymers attaining sizes of several million daltons. The ECM is composed of proteins and carbohydrate polymers which are secreted into the space between the cells and which are likely to contribute to the higher organisation structure of the ECM by interacting with each other and with the surfaces of the cells. The interactions of the molecules of the ECM with the membrane-bound receptors on the cell surface, provides structural coherence to the organisation of the tissue, and a means of transmitting extracellular signals into the cells, or alternatively of sending signals from cells via molecules in the ECM (Figure 1).

In general, the biological response involves multiple cellular interactions with individual ECM molecules and with multiple sites within the same molecule. Many ECM proteins form large families with some 30 genes identified for collagens and 12 identified for laminins. The biological activity of the ECM has been studied in vitro using either complex three-dimensional matrices (either cell- or tissue-derived), or individual components (purified proteins, proteolytic or recombinant fragments of ECM components, or peptides) that have been used as immobilised plated substrates or added to the culture medium (Garwood et al., 2001; Cukierman et al., 2002; Garwood et al., 2002). Laminin has been the most vigorously studied ECM molecule using this approach and more than 40 active sites for specific functions have been defined (Colognato et al., 2002; Li et al., 2002). However, additional complexity can be found in ECM molecules at other levels. Alternative splicing of mRNA transcripts can generate a variety of isoforms for many ECM proteins and their receptors. For example, Tenascin-C in mouse has up to 64 possible isoforms of which 27 have been characterised in mouse brain (Joester & Faissner, 1999). Further variety can also be obtained by proteolytic processing which may release active sites or expose "cryptic" active sites. Many ECM molecules contain such cryptic active sites that are released or become available as a result of such processing. For example, cleavage of laminin during mammary gland involution releases a fragment that binds to the epidermal growth factor (EGF) receptor and increases cell migration (Schenk et al., 2003). Similarly, the anti-angiogenic molecules, endostatin and tumstatin, are degraded products of collagen XVIII and collagen IV, respectively (Sudhakar et al., 2003). These cryptic sites, as well as the active sites, relate to in vivo functions in development and during remodeling. The addition of glycosylation by post-translational modification can also significantly change the nature of ECM proteins. For example, the oligosaccharides HNK-1 (sulfated glucuronic acid), and Lewis-X (sialyl-Lewis-X) on phosphacan (Garwood et al., 1999), which have been implicated in IgCAM interactions (Milev et al., 1997) and neural cell migration. Through such mechanisms the number of unique structures in the ECM can be increased and the functions of these large, multifunctional molecules expanded. Historically, the ECM was thought of as a mechanical structure, necessary for the physical delimitation of tissues. However, ECMs not only provide support, tensile strength and scaffolding for tissues and cells, but also serve as three-dimensional substructures for cell adhesion and movement, as a storage depot for growth factors, chemokines and cytokines, and as signals for morphogenesis and differentiation (Figure 1).

The biological responses to the ECM are regulated by specific cell-surface receptors (Ruoslahti, 1996; Chothia & Jones, 1997; Peles *et al.*, 1998; Garwood *et al.*, 2002). Multiple ECM signals transmitted via diverse surface receptors are integrated by intracellular signalling pathways to affect the cellular response. Many different receptors have been identified that transduce signals to the cytoskeleton and nucleus. These include members of the heterodimeric integrins (Ruoslahti, 1996), receptor tyrosine kinases (Hubbard, 1999) and tyrosine phosphatases (Zhang, 1998), immunogloblulin superfamily receptors (Chothia & Jones, 1997), and cell-surface proteoglycans (Carey, 1997). Since a given ECM molecule may actively interact with a number of different receptors, the complexity of potential cell-ECM interactions is enormous and may be affected by the relative localised concentrations of particular forms of ECM molecules and the availability of their active sites, together with the actual repertoire of cell-surface receptors for ECM signals expressed by a particular cell type at a particular developmental stage. For example, on laminin-1, some 40 active sites have been identified and these can be recognised by at least 20 different receptors (Kleinman *et al.*, 2003).

The importance of ECM molecules in development has been proven by in vivo studies using gene targeting (Gustafsson & Fassler, 2000). Mice lacking certain ECM component genes die before birth, whereas others survive and exhibit unique tissue phenotypes.

NEURAL ECM, STEM CELL NICHE, AND DIFFERENTIATION OF PRECURSOR CELL POPULATIONS

In the central nervous system (CNS), as in other tissues, the fundamental properties of self-renewal and multipotency (generating neurons and the glial cell types: astrocytes, and oligodendrocytes) are retained by neural stem cells throughout life. However, the problems of limited regeneration of CNS neurons and their functional networks following injury highlight some of the considerable challenges facing the search for therapeutic solutions to neurological diseases and lesions.

Stem cells are localised in several discrete regions of the CNS (Alvarez-Buylla *et al.*, 2001; Doetsch, 2003). During brain development, neuroepithelial stem cells located in the ventricular zone next to the ventricles give rise to neurons and glia. Although neurogenesis is mostly complete by birth, gliogenesis continues throughout life. However, two germinal regions persist in the adult mammalian brain that generate large numbers of neurons: the subventricular zone (SVZ) and the subgranular zone of the hippocampal formation. In other words, the developmental programme of neural stem cells results in their restriction to localised regions of the CNS and a switch in the major cell type produced by the stem cells from neurons to glia (Kilpatrick & Bartlett, 1995; Qian *et al.*, 2000; Alvarez-Buylla *et al.*, 2001). This developmental programme of the neural stem cells appears to be regulated by both intrinsic and extrinsic factors. The observation that single stem cells grown in culture give rise first to neurons and then later to glia in sequential cell divisions points to intrinsic timing mechanisms regulating the fate of the daughter cells (Qian *et al.*, 2000). On the other hand, growth factors and cytokines can strongly affect the development of stem cells pointing to the existence of extrinsic mechanisms, for example, bFGF (FGF2) can promote the expression of the EGF receptor (EGF-R) on neural stem cells, while by contrast, bone morphogenic protein 4 (BMP4) inhibits EGF-R expression (Ciccolini & Svendsen, 1998; Lillien & Raphael, 2000).

At the present time, the best-studied factors regulating neural stem cell behaviour are the growth factors. Epidermal growth factor (EGF), basic fibroblast growth factor (FGF2) and transforming growth factor alpha (TGFα) are mitogens for neural stem cells both in vivo and in vitro (Kilpatrick & Bartlett, 1995). Other growth factors including bone morphogenic proteins (BMPs), platelet-derived growth factor (PDGF), ciliary neurotrophic factor (CNTF) and brain-derived neurotrophic factor (BDNF) can regulate stem cell differentiation (Gross *et al.*, 1996; Johe *et al.*, 1996; Benoit *et al.*, 2001). The timing of growth factor responses reflects a changing pattern of growth factor receptor expression during neural stem cell development, driven, at least in part, by the growth factors themselves. Early embryonic neural stem cells respond only to FGF2 whereas late embryonic and adult neural stem cells are responsive to both FGF2 and EGF (Kilpatrick & Bartlett, 1995; Burrows *et al.*, 1997; Alvarez-Buylla & Temple, 1998; Qian *et al.*, 2000), with the acquisition of EGF responsiveness stimulated by FGF2 and inhibited by BMP4 (Lillien & Raphael, 2000). The BMPs have been shown to promote proliferation, apoptosis or terminal differentiation of neural stem cells into either neurons or glial cells at progressively later stages of embryonic development (Gross *et al.*, 1996) (Panchision *et al.*, 2001). During the expansion phase of neural stem cell development, precursor cells express BMPR1A and respond to BMP by proliferation and by upregulation of a second BMP receptor, BMPR1B. This receptor triggers mitotic arrest once levels exceed that of BMPR1A, so initiating the differentiation phase of neural stem cell development (Panchision *et al.*, 2001).

In vivo, these combined mechanisms ensure that gliogenesis follows a period of neurogenesis in CNS development whilst maintaining a population of stem cells in the developing CNS that will subsequently persist throughout adult life (Alvarez-Buylla & Temple, 1998; Alvarez-Buylla *et al.*, 2001). As development proceeds and the CNS becomes a complex three-dimensional structure, the neural stem cells that generate all three major cell lineages in the CNS, neurons, astrocytes and oligodendrocytes, become restricted to the specialised germinal zones, particularly the ventricular zone (VZ) in embryonic development, and the sub-ventricular zone (SVZ) in later embryonic and the postnatal CNS, with the latter persisting throughout adult life (Gates *et al.*, 1995; Doetsch *et al.*, 1997). Within these regions, which are analogous to the stem cell niches described in other tissues, stem cells divide either to increase the size of the neural stem cell pool or to generate committed precursor cells for neural or glial cell lineages. These different daughter cell populations appear to be generated largely sequentially, with an expansion phase followed by neurogenesis and then gliogenesis (Temple, 2001).

At the same time, the cellular identities of the neural stem cells themselves appears to change, and are currently thought to be found within a lineage encompassing neuroepithelial cells, radial glial cells and astrocytes, all of which show stem cell properties at different developmental stages (Alvarez-Buylla *et al.*, 2001; Doetsch, 2003). However, the mechanisms that regulate these stem cell developmental programmes within the microenvironments of the VZ and SVZ are incompletely understood, and are important not only because of their central role in CNS development, but also because an understanding of the mechanisms underlying the expansion and differentiation of neural stem cells is important for therapeutic strategies based on cell replacement.

The soluble and diffusible properties of growth factors make them capable of signalling over a long range. The restricted localization of neural stem cells in embryonic and postnatal development, and their developmental regulation independent of adjacent regions of the CNS, therefore suggests the presence of mechanisms whose role is to restrict or amplify growth factor signalling. One such mechanism is the secretion of short-range inhibitory factors such as the BMP inhibitor, noggin. The production of noggin by ependymal cells prevents adjacent neural stem cells from responding to the gliogenic properties of BMPs in the adult mouse SVZ, so generating a restricted neurogenic environment (Lim *et al.*, 2000). Another potential mechanism is the distribution of extracellular matrix (ECM) molecules. One of these, Tenascin C (TN-C), is highly expressed within the SVZ throughout postnatal and adult life (Gates *et al.*, 1995).

Tenascin-C – An Example of an ECM Molecule That Has Effects on the Development in the CNS of Stem Cell and Precursor Cell Populations

Tenascin-C is a large glycoprotein displaying many of the characteristics of ECM proteins, including a modular structure, extensive isoform variation, proteolytic processing, and selective modification by glycosylation. TN-C is highly expressed in the SVZ of the CNS throughout life and has been found to be prominently expressed by neural stem cells.

Structure of Tenascin-C

Tenascins are characterised by a serial arrangement of a cysteine-rich amino-terminus, followed by varying numbers of epidermal growth factor-type repeats (EGF), succeeded by multiple fibronectin type III repeats (FNIII), and a carboxy-terminus with homologies to fibrinogen-beta and –gamma (Jones & Jones, 2000a; Jones & Jones, 2000b; Joester & Faissner, 2001) (Figure 2).

The basic TN-C protein in mouse comprises 14.5 EGF-type repeats, followed by 8 FNIII repeats. However, there is considerable splicing of upto six additional FNIII domains between the fifth and sixth FNIII units of the basic structure, potentially resulting in upto 64 different isoforms, of which 27 have been shown to be expressed as mRNAs (Joester & Faissner, 1999).

TN-C monomers range in size between 190 and 300 kDa but it seems likely that they occur as disulfide-linked oligomers. Rotary shadowing images show that, in vitro, TN-C forms a striking, highly symmetrical structure called a hexabrachion. The six monomer chains are linked at their amino termini via a tenascin assembly (TA) domain which contains cysteine residues and between 3 and 4 alpha-helical heptad repeats that enable the amino termini of TN polypeptides to be linked into oligomeric structures. Assembly of the TN-C hexabrachion is a two-step process, involving formation of trimers and then linkage of trimers into hexamers. Trimer formation is initiated by association of three TN-C polypeptides in a triple-stranded coiled coil by the heptad repeats. Trimers are further stabilized by inter-chain disulfide bonds at two cysteine residues amino terminal to the heptad region. The clustering of TN-C chains creates a multivalent TA domain that interacts homophilically with another trimer to form a hexamer. Hexamers are then stabilized by

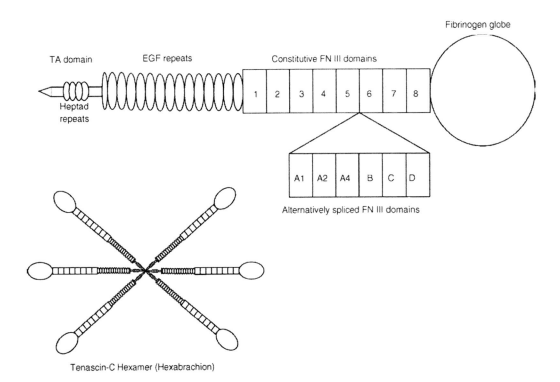

Figure 2. The Structure Of Tenascin-C.

The modular structure of mouse TN-C is shown, consisting of 14.5 EGF repeats and 8 FN III domains in the basic protein. Alternative splicing between FN III 5 and 6 can result in the addition of upto another six FN III domains. In human TN-C, there are upto 9 alternatively spliced FN III domains. The representation of the TN-C hexamer or hexabrachion is based on rotary shadowing images of the purified protein.

disulfide linkages at a cysteine residue that is located 50 residues amino terminal to the heptad repeat (Jones & Jones, 2000a; Jones & Jones, 2000b). TN-C is also capable of forming nonamers, indicating that native TN-C molecules exist predominantly as multiples of three. Heterotypic hexamers have been observed in which a trimer containing a particular variant of TN-C is linked to a trimer containing a different variant.

The fibronectin type III domains contain approximately 90 amino acids and are extended globular structures composed of seven antiparallel beta-strands arranged in two sheets. FNIII arrays are highly elastic and can be stretched to several times their length and refolded rapidly. Particular peptide motifs within individual FNIII domains bind to several ligands including other ECM proteins, glycosaminoglycans, and a number of different cell surface receptors. FNIII domains are susceptible to proteolytic degradation, allowing TN-C-containing matrices to be selectively remodeled, particularly by matrix metalloproteinases (MMPs) and serine proteases (Jones & Jones, 2000a; Jones & Jones, 2000b). The nature and number of FNIII domains in TN-C polypeptides are altered by alternative RNA splicing. This can generate a considerable diversity in the functions of TN-C polypeptides. Thus, in mouse, there are six spliced FNIII domains, whereas in human TN-C, at least nine different FNIII domains have been identified that are differentially included or excluded by RNA splicing.

Some of the TN-C splice variants occur at distinct frequencies during development of the nervous system, in smooth muscle, kidney, and the cornea. Using RT-PCR, as many as 27 different FNIII variants of TN-C have been found during mouse brain development, indicating that many of the theoretically possible combinations of FNIII repeats are likely to be expressed during tissue morphogenesis. Selection of particular TN-C splice variants is modulated by the proliferative state of the cell, by extracellular pH, and by polypeptide growth factors such as TGF-beta1. Currently, however, the mechanisms that determine preferential splice site selection of TN-C mRNAs in the region of the FNIII repeats are unknown (Jones & Jones, 2000a; Jones & Jones, 2000b; Joester & Faissner, 2001).

TN-C occurs as a glycoprotein with upto 20 N-glycosylation sites in the full-length isoform. Enzymatic digestion of TN-C with N-glycosidase F reduces its apparent size on SDS-PAGE by around 20-30 kD. Interestingly a disproportionate number of the N-glycosylation sites occur in the alternatively spliced FNIII domains: there are 3 sites on the 8 constitutive FNIII domains but upto 11 sites are present in the spliced domains. The differential addition of sugars with additional functions, such as the HNK-1 epitope, which is implicated in neural cell migration, is another level at which the properties of TN-C protein may be altered (Garwood et al., 2001).

The fibrinogen globe contains polypeptide loops formed by two consecutive intrachain disulfide bonds. It can bind calcium through an EF-hand motif and this calcium-binding property can also influence interactions with other proteins (Jones & Jones, 2000a; Jones & Jones, 2000b).

Tenascin-C Expression In Vivo

TN-C is prominent in embryonic and adult tissues that are actively remodeling (Jones & Jones, 2000b; Chiquet-Ehrismann & Chiquet, 2003). TN-C expression can be correlated with key events of neurohistogenesis, such as cell proliferation in the ventricular and subventricular zones, neuronal migration, segregation of neuronal assemblies and extension of neuronal processes.

In the CNS, TN-C is widely expressed during early development and is then progressively downregulated during further differentiation of the tissue (Faissner, 1997; Garwood et al., 2001). There is little or no expression of TN-C in fully developed organs (Chiquet-Ehrismann & Chiquet, 2003), but in the adult CNS, TN-C expression remains adjacent to areas of active neurogenesis such as the hippocampus and the borders of the subventricular zone (Miragall et al., 1990; Bartsch et al., 1992; Gates et al., 1995; Jankovski & Sotelo, 1996). However, TN-C is actively re-expressed in the adult brain under pathological conditions such as infection, inflammation, lesioning, or tumorigenesis (Crossin, 1996; Deller et al., 1997; Garwood et al., 2001; Heck et al., 2004).

Overall, these expression patterns suggest important roles for TN-C in the modulation of cell behaviour during periods of active CNS modelling and plasticity, an observation supported by functional studies which show that TN-C can significantly alter CNS cell behaviour, often in a cell type-specific manner (Faissner & Kruse, 1990; Taylor et al., 1993; Faissner & Steindler, 1995).

TN-C is mainly produced by glia in the developing CNS, for example, along radial and Bergmann glial fibers during neuronal migration in the cortex and cerebellum (Bartsch et al.,

1992; Husmann *et al.*, 1992). It has also been found to be expressed on some types of neuron, such as discrete populations of cortical and thalamic neurons (Kusakabe *et al.*, 2001). However, its expression on precursor cell populations has been less well characterised. In rodents, a distinct expression of TN-C is observed in the developing subventricular zone. For example, at E17, there is some punctate staining in the dorsolateral SVZ but most of the observed immunostaining is extracellular throughout the proliferative zones (Gates *et al.*, 1995). A lateral-to-medial and caudorostral gradient of TN-C protein has been found in the late embryonic and early postnatal striatum (O'Brien *et al.*, 1992). Double-labeling studies have shown that immature glia and radial glia are the main cells in the dorsal SVZ expressing TN-C transcripts at P3, while in the adult it seems to be mostly GFAP+ astrocytes. However, given the possibility of different subsets of migrating neurons and glia displaying a variety of orientations, it was noted that a certain degree of interpretation was required regarding which cell or morphogenetic events each of the markers may have identified (Gates *et al.*, 1995; Gotz *et al.*, 1997; Kusakabe *et al.*, 2001).

In vitro, TN-C expression has also been shown on OPCs (Garwood *et al.*, 2004) and an extensive gene expression profiling study of neural stem cells in 8 day neurospheres found TN-C to be the most highly expressed gene of the 2458 gene transcripts that were identified (Ramalho-Santos *et al.*, 2002).

Tenascin-C Structure/Function Studies In Vitro: Cell Adhesion, Cell Migration, Cellular Process Outgrowth

TN-C is an ECM protein in the developing CNS that can affect diverse aspects of cell behaviour. Unlike a classical, universal adhesion protein such as fibronectin, TN-C can have contrasting effects on different cell types. Consequently, in the same experimental set-up, TN-C may be adhesive and promigratory for one cell type, but inhibitory for another, and the effect of TN-C on a single cell type may vary depending on the cell's contact with other ECM components and on the mode of presentation of the protein (Jones & Jones, 2000b; Garwood *et al.*, 2001; Chiquet-Ehrismann & Chiquet, 2003).

TN-C has been shown in different in vitro assays to exert both inhibitory and stimulatory actions on neuronal cells affecting cell adhesion and migration, and axon growth and guidance (Husmann *et al.*, 1992; Meiners *et al.*, 1995; Gotz *et al.*, 1996; Deller *et al.*, 1997; Faissner, 1997; Gotz *et al.*, 1997). These diverse functions have been localised to distinct functional domains using proteolytic fragments and fusion proteins (Figure 3). Hence, for example, an analysis of the alternatively spliced FNIII domains shows that together they support short-term, but not long-term, adhesion of embryonic and early post-natal neurons, whilst FNIII domains A1, A2, and A4 together exhibit repulsive properties on hippocampal neurons, whereas FNIII BD and D6 promote neurite-outgrowth (Gotz *et al.*, 1996; Rigato *et al.*, 2002). These contrary cellular functions also seem to depend on their mode of presentation, that is, whether the proteins are soluble or substrate-bound, and also upon the cell types and differentiation states of the target tissues (Gotz *et al.*, 1997).

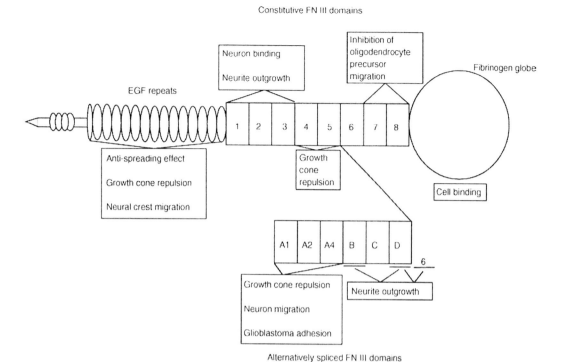

Figure 3. Structure-Function Assignments Of Tenascin-C Domains Based On In Vitro Assays Of Neural Cells.

The combined application of monoclonal antibodies, perturbation studies, and the use of recombinant protein constructs resulted in the localisation of different functions to distinct parts of the molecule (Garwood et al. 2001).

Antibody blocking studies with specific monoclonal antibodies show that these multiple functions of TN-C are associated with different sites on the molecule. Thus, an antibody which blocks neurite outgrowth promotion by TN-C was not efficient in blocking the anti-adhesive properties of the glycoprotein, nor its influence on oligodendrocyte precursor motility (Lochter *et al.*, 1991; Frost *et al.*, 1996; Kiernan *et al*, 1996).

To further analyse the differential properties of the different domains of TN-C, fusion proteins have been expressed and purified from bacterial and mammalian expression systems and the resulting constructs have been tested in *in vitro* bioassays. Thus, a cell binding site for cerebellar neurons could be attributed to the FNIII-domains 1-3 while a neurite outgrowth promoting site could be attributed to FNIII-repeats, BD and D6 around the distal splice site of TN-C (Gotz *et al.*, 1996). Using analogous methods, the site responsible for the inhibition of oligodendrocyte precursor migration could be attributed to the FN domains 7,8 (Kiernan *et al.*, 1996). A summary of functions ascribed to the different domains of TN-C is shown in Figure 3.

However, in addition to adhesive effects, there is increasing evidence that TN-C can modulate the cell cycle, affecting proliferation, growth, morphological differentiation, and cell survival.

Tenascin-C Knockout Studies In Vivo: Cell Proliferation, Regulation Of Growth Factor Signalling, Morphological Differentiation, Cell Survival

A number of observations suggest that TN-C may play an important general role in stem cell niches as a modulator of growth factor signalling (Garcion *et al.*, 2001; Garcion *et al.*, 2004; Garwood *et al.*, 2004). TN-C-deficient mice have altered numbers of different neural stem cell populations, with a reduction in the number of radial glia and oligodendrocyte precursor cells (Garcion *et al.*, 2001; Garcion *et al.*, 2004), and an increase in FGF-responsive progenitor cells, that have an increased probability of generating neurons when grown in cell culture (Garcion *et al.*, 2004). In addition, an inhibition of hematopoesis in the TN-C knockout indicates effects on other stem and precursor cell populations (Ohta *et al.*, 1998).

NEURAL STEM CELLS AND THE TN-C KNOCKOUT

Studies of the effects of an absence of TN-C on neural stem cell development have found that there are significant differences in the responses of stem cells in the TN-C knockout to growth factors compared to wild-type littermates (Figure 4). Stem cells in the embryonic mammalian CNS are initially responsive to fibroblast growth factor 2 (FGF2). They then undergo a developmental programme in which they acquire epidermal growth factor (EGF) responsiveness, switch from the production of neuronal to glial precursors and become localized in specialized germinal zones such as the subventricular zone (SVZ). The acquisition of the EGF receptor (EGF-R) is delayed in TN-C knockout mice (Garcion *et al.*, 2004). While wild-type mice had acquired the EGF-R in the SVZ by E12.5, EGF-R was not observed in the TN-C knockout until E17.5. It could be shown that this delayed acquisition of EGF-R in vivo was reflected by numerous differences in the behaviour of neurospheres derived from these stem cell populations. Wild-type neurospheres from E10.5 grew in response to FGF2 (that is, they were FGF-responsive) and a proportion also grew in response to EGF (that is, were already EGF-responsive). However, none of the neural stem cells from the TN-C knockout embryos were EGF-responsive.

This lack of response to EGF could be correlated to differences in EGF-R expression in the TN-C knockout: at E10.5, wild-type neurospheres expressed EGF-R when grown in FGF2; however, no EGF-R was detected in TN-C knockout neurospheres even after 5 days growth in the presence of FGF2. Significantly, this phenotype could be rescued by addition of exogenous TN-C protein to the culture, resulting in EGF-R expression in the TN-C knockout spheres. A further analysis of the response of TN-C knockout neurospheres (from E12.5 and P0) to FGF2 showed that they proliferated less than wild-type spheres (Garcion *et al.*, 2004).

Overall, these results indicate that EGF-R expression in neural stem cells is delayed by the absence of TN-C. Since it has been shown that EGF-R expression in neural stem cell populations can be stimulated by FGF2 but inhibited by another growth factor, BMP4, it was postulated that such responses would be altered in TN-C knockout cells. Although EGF-R expression was found in both TN-C knockout and wild-type neurospheres (from E12.5 and P0) after 3 days growth in FGF2, this expression of EGF-R could be inhibited by BMP4 much more efficiently in TN-C knockout cells, indicating that TN-C normally functions as an inhibitor of BMP4 signalling, thereby enhancing EGF-R expression (Figure 4).

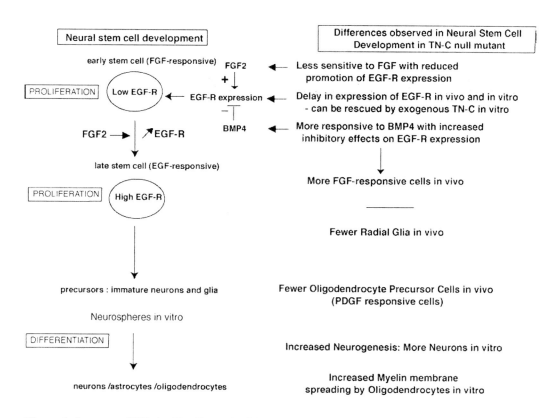

Figure 4. Summary Of Roles For Tenascin-C In Neural Stem Cell Development Based On Studies Of TN-C Knockout Mice

On the left-hand side is a schema showing the transition from an early, FGF-responsive stem cell to a late, EGF-responsive stem cell, with the acquisition of the EGF receptor (EGF-R). On the right-hand side, the main effects on this process observed in the TN-C knockout are described, highlighting changes in the response of TN-C deficient stem cells to FGF2 and BMP4. The further development of the late stem cells into precursors and their differentiation into mature cell types is also affected in the TN-C knockout with an increase in neurogenesis from TN-C-deficient neurospheres and multiple effects on the oligodendroglial lineage (see Figure 5) (Garcion et al. 2001, 2004; Garwood et al. 2004).

By plating neural stem cells at clonal density in the presence of FGF2, it could be shown that there were more FGF2-responsive neurospheres derived from the TN-C knockout than wild-type mice (although TN-C spheres were smaller), indicating that the TN-C-deficient CNS contains more FGF2-responsive neural stem cells than wild-type CNS (Garcion *et al.*, 2004).

In order to study the effects of the absence of TN-C upon the formation of neurons and glia, the neurospheres were allowed to differentiate by plating onto poly-lysine substrate. The adherent cells differentiated into neurons, astrocytes, and oligodendrocytes, with more neurons being formed from TN-C knockout spheres. This increase in neurogenesis was observed for striatum-derived neurospheres grown in either FGF2 or EGF, but was only observed for cortex-derived spheres grown in EGF. Addition of exogneous TN-C protein to

FGF2 stimulated TN-C knockout spheres rescued the phenotype, reversing the increase in neurogenesis.

Although no quantitative differences were observed in relative levels of gliogenesis in TN-C knockout neurospheres, qualitative differences were observed in the differentiation of oligodendrocytes (discussed in the next section).

Overall this study showed that TN-C can facilitate normal neural stem cell development by modulating the sensitivity of neural stem cells to the two growth factors, FGF2 and BMP4, that regulate EGF-R expression. TN-C enhances sensitivity to FGF2 and decreases sensitivity to BMP4. Several potential mechanisms exist by which these effects of TN-C could be mediated. An extracellular interaction of the growth factors with TN-C could inhibit or potentiate its effect, as seen with the interaction between FGF and heparan sulphate proteoglycans (Carey, 1997). Alternatively, TN-C could interact with a specific cell surface receptor, and intracellular components of the signalling pathway downstream of this TN-C receptor could then interact with growth factor receptor signalling pathways (Jones & Jones, 2000b), as was shown for oligodendrocyte precursor cells in the TN-C null mouse (Garcion et al., 2001). Finally, TN-C could regulate intracellular signalling by the interaction with cell surface phosphatases such as members of the receptor protein tyrosine phosphatase family, which could then in turn regulate the activity of intracellular kinases (Milev et al., 1997).

The observed effects of TN-C on neural stem cell development also suggest that TN-C is one of the factors regulating transitions to successive stem cell developmental stages that are dependent upon growth factor signalling (in this case, FGF2 and BMP4) consistent with a "fast-forward" model of neural stem cell development. In this respect, both BMP and FGF2 have been shown to promote proliferation of a particular stage of neural stem cell development and the expression of the next growth factor receptor in the developmental progression, the BMPR1B receptor and the EGF-R, respectively (Lillien & Raphael, 2000; Panchision et al., 2001). Once these receptors reach a threshold level, signalling is initiated and the transition to the next developmental stage is made. Neural stem cells from TN-C knockout mice show reduced sensitivity to the effects of FGF2, and this reduced sensitivity inhibits EGF-R expression and subsequent entry into the EGF-responsive stem cell compartment. This would have the effect of expanding the FGF-responsive stem cell population undergoing self-renewing divisions in their compartment (which require lower levels of FGF2 signalling) and could explain the higher numbers of FGF-responsive stem cells observed in the TN-C knockout mice.

TN-C deficiency also has effects on the number of radial glia, another neural stem cell population (Hartfuss et al., 2001). However, in contrast to the effects on FGF-responsive cells, there was a significant reduction in the numbers of radial glia observed in TN-C knockout mice at E13.5, E18.5, and P0, although the morphology of these RC2-positive cells was unchanged. The precise relationships between radial glia, neurosphere-forming cells and EGF-responsive neural stem cells are unknown, although radial glia do develop from the original neuroepithelium so their reduction in the TNC-deficient mice could also be consistent with a role for TN-C in promoting the developmental progression by which the neural stem cells of the neuroepithelium alter both growth factor sensitivity and cellular identity. In this model a critical function for TNC is therefore the acceleration of the feed-forward mechanism and this may be one role for the observed maintenance of expression of TN-C in the postnatal SVZ (Gates et al., 1995), so providing an environment that facilitates the production and differentiation of precursor cells when required in response to injury or cell loss. In addition, the expression of TN-C by the radial glial cells themselves (Gotz *et al.*, 1998) and the observation from gene expression profiling studies that TN-C is very highly enriched in 8-day-old neurospheres (Ramalho-Santos *et al.*, 2002) shows that TN-C is produced by neural stem cells or their progeny, and may therefore provide an autocrine/paracrine factor in a positive feedback loop for neural stem cell development.

Oligodendrocyte Precursor Cells And TN-C

Studies of TN-C knockout mice have also revealed effects of an absence of TN-C upon precursor cells populations in the CNS, particularly oligodendrocyte precursor cells (OPCs) (Garcion *et al.*, 2001; Garwood *et al.*, 2004). A summary of these effects is shown in Figure 5.

Oligodendrocyte precursor cells (OPCs) are neural cells that are particularly sensitive to environmental cues for their normal development. They are generated in restricted areas of the developing CNS out of which they migrate, sometimes over considerable distances (Levison *et al.*, 1993; Ono *et al.*, 1995), to their final destinations, where they differentiate into mature, myelin-forming oligodendrocytes (Miller, 2002). Most of this development occurs postnatally when neuronal pathways are already established; hence, localised interactions between OPCs and cellular and extracellular cues that they encounter are critical in determining their fate (Blaschuk *et al.*, 2000; Colognato *et al.*, 2002; Miller, 2002). OPCs are proliferative, migratory, bipolar cells that are identified by their expression of gangliosides reacting with the monoclonal antibody A2B5. These cells proliferate in response to a number of growth factors including FGF2 and platelet-derived growth factor (PDGF) (Bogler *et al.*, 1990; Tang *et al.*, 2000). In the absence of mitogens, OPCs immediately stop dividing and can follow a bipotential fate in culture, since they are capable of differentiation into either oligodendrocytes or into type-2 astrocytes and have therefore been also called oligodendrocyte type-2 astrocyte (O-2A) progenitor cells (Raff *et al.*, 1983). Differentiation into oligodendrocytes appears to be the favoured pathway, occurring rapidly in a chemically defined, serum-free medium containing thyroid hormones (Raff *et al.*, 1983; Vos *et al.*, 1996).

In the TN-C knockout mice, an overall reduction in the levels of cell proliferation (measured by BrdU incorporation) was observed in the SVZ at postnatal ages (P0 to P17) (Garcion *et al.*, 2001). Only a small proportion of these cells were OPCs (NG2-positive) in the TN-C knockout compared to wild-type indicating that TN-C deficiency results in a reduction in OPC proliferation. This lower rate of proliferation in the TN-C knockout was confirmed in vitro with OPC primary cultures, and it could be shown that the TN-C knockout OPCs were insensitive to the mitogenic effects of PDGF. Addition of exogenous TN-C protein to the TN-C-deficient substrate rescued this phenotype, restoring the response to PDGF of both TN-C-deficient and wild-type OPCs grown on TN-C deficient substrates, although wild-type OPCs remained two-fold more responsive to the mitogenic effect of PDGF. Further investigation of the promotion by exogenous TN-C protein of the mitogenic effects of PDGF on OPCs showed that TN-C was acting via an integrin receptor (αVβ3): use of a function-blocking monoclonal antibody against the integrin abolished the TN-C mediated effect. This is particularly interesting in the light of the subsequent discovery that

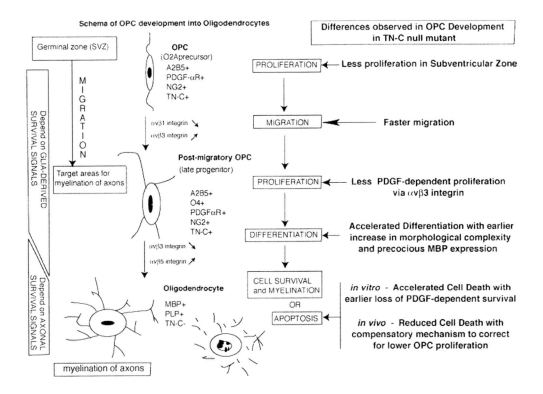

Figure 5. Summary Of The Principal Aspects Of OPC Development Illustrating Differences Observed For Tn-C Knockout OPCs In Vivo And In Vitro.

Highly migratory, proliferating OPCs are generated in the subventricular zone of the lateral ventricles. These cells express antigenic markers such as A2B5, NG2, and the PDGF-a receptor. In vivo, these cells migrate to the zones of myelination where they undergo a final stage of proliferation (O4-positive) before terminal differentiation into oligodendrocytes (expression of myelin components such as MBP and PLP). TN-C expression corresponds to the precursor stages (A2B5 and O4-positive). A change in integrin receptor dimer composition on OPCs accompanies these different cell stages: $\alpha v \beta 1$ downregulation coincides with loss of the migratory phenotype; $\alpha v \beta 3$ integrin is expressed by post-migratory OPCs and then downregulated when these cells differentiate into oligodendrocytes (with the corresponding upregulation of $\alpha v \beta 5$ integrin). In the TN-C knockout OPCs proliferate less, migrate faster, and are less sensitive to the mitogenic effects of PDGF. Subsequently, TN-C knockout OPCs display an accelerated differentiation into oligodendrocytes with the precocious appearance of MBP and earlier promotion of process elaboration. In vitro, the faster development of post-migratory TN-C knockout OPCs towards terminal differentiation into oligodendrocytes results in increased levels of apoptosis and earlier loss of response to the survival effects of PDGF, possibly due to a switch in the repertoire of survival factors from dependence on glia-derived factors such as PDGF towards axonal-derived survival signals. In vitro, TN-C knockout OPCs die more rapidly in the absence of neuronal survival factors. However, in vivo, axonal-derived survival signals are still present in the TN-C knockout, reducing oligodendrocyte apoptosis in zones of myelination, and serving as a compensatory mechanism to correct for the reduction in the size of the TN-C knockout OPC population. This hypothesis is supported by observation of equivalent numbers of oligodendrocytes developing from TN-C knockout and wild-type neurospheres (Garcion et al. 2001; Garwood et al. 2004).

there is an endogenous expression of TN-C by wild-type OPCs, since it indicates that there are mechanisms of TN-C action on OPCs which require its presence in the ECM substrate and that this cannot be readily compensated for by an endogenous production of TN-C protein (Garwood et al., 2004).

In fact, by RT-PCR analysis of OPCs prepared from neonatal mice, it was found that OPCs were capable of expressing transcripts for TN-C isoforms covering the entire size range from the shortest TN-C isoform (with no additional FNIII inserts) to the largest isoform (with all of the additional FNIII domains inserted), suggesting that OPCs have the capacity to produce TN-C protein monomers from the shortest to the largest isoform (Garwood et al., 2004). These results suggest that an extensive heterogeneity in the expression of TN-C isoforms is possible within a single cell type and tend to reinforce the proposition that TN-C expression is subject to complex variations in dynamically localised microenvironments (Jones & Jones, 2000a; Jones & Jones, 2000b; Garwood et al., 2001; Joester & Faissner, 2001). The mechanisms by which TN-C affects OPC development remain to be determined but it seems likely that endogenous expression of TN-C by OPCs could modulate the regulatory effects of TN-C that we have characterised by introducing a possible autocrine response. OPCs traverse relatively long distances in the developing CNS and are exposed to exogenous sources of TN-C, especially TN-C secreted by astrocytes. The capacity of OPCs to endogenously express a range of TN-C isoforms could contribute to a dynamic modulation of their immediate extracellular environment, adjusting their cellular responses under certain conditions. Such a paracrine/autocrine mechanism for endogenous TN-C effects on proliferation and process elongation in astrocyte development has also recently been proposed (Nishio et al., 2003). However, in addition to the range of specific TN-C isoforms that may be produced by a given cell type under given conditions, changes in the binding specificity and the temporal repertoire of potential TN-C receptors, for example, integrins, expressed during OPC development and differentiation may also affect the response of OPCs to TN-C (Garcion et al., 2001). Thus, TN-C can control cell behaviour both indirectly by binding other matrix components and also directly by interactions with specific cell surface receptors (Jones & Jones, 2000b).

As a substrate for OPCs, TN-C has been shown to be anti-adhesive and inhibitory for OPC migration in vitro (Frost et al., 1996; Kiernan et al., 1996), and analysis of the TN-C knockout mice reveals faster migration of OPCs out of the germinal zones in vivo, with an earlier appearance of OPCs in zones of future myelination, for example, in the neonatal optic nerve and at points nearer the retina of the knockout mice compared to wild-type (Garcion et al., 2001).

However, in addition to displaying faster migration, TN-C knockout OPCs display precocious differentiation. When grown in culture in the absence of growth factor stimulation, OPCs from the TN-C knockout expressed the myelin basic protein (MBP) after 48 hours while a similar MBP expression was not observed in wild-type OPCs before 96 hours (Garwood et al., 2004). The morphology of TN-C knockout OPCs changed more rapidly from the bipolar precursor to a multiprocessed one with longer process formation and branching than the wild-type. Differences in the subcellular localisation of the PDGF α receptor (PDGF-R), and the tyrosine phosphatase receptor, RPTP-beta, that can bind TN-C, were also observed in the TN-C knockout OPCs. Similarly, the more extensive differentiation of TN-C deficient oligodendrocytes was observed in differentiated neurospheres prepared from TN-C knockout mice. Although the proportion of oligodendrocytes (MBP/Gal-C positive) in both TN-C knockout and wild-type spheres was the same at around 2%, the oligodendrocytes in the absence of TN-C had longer processes and there was more extensive myelin membrane formation, as indicated by the degree of cell spreading of TN-C knockout oligodendrocytes (Garwood *et al.*, 2004).

The last aspect of OPC development considered was cell survival versus apoptosis. There is normally a large excess production of OPCs in the CNS compared to the final number of oligodendrocytes that end up myelinating axons. In vivo, it seems that oligodendroglial survival signals come from an interplay between glial-derived components (including PDGF, LIF, and CNTF), and the non-myelinated axons (Barres & Raff, 1999; Casaccia-Bonnefil, 2000). Hence, although proliferative, migratory OPCs respond to glia-derived factors, mature oligodendrocytes depend on axonal signals for long-term survival (Trapp *et al.*, 1997; Barres & Raff, 1999): for example, laminin-2 on the axonal surface promotes survival of newly generated oligodendrocytes via the $\alpha6\beta1$ integrin (Frost *et al.*, 1999; Colognato *et al.*, 2002). From our studies, TN-C may serve as an oligodendroglial survival factor by maintaining OPCs in a less differentiated proliferative state. A much higher rate of apoptosis was observed in cultures of TN-C knockout OPCs (60% TUNEL-positive cells after 24 hours) compared to wild-type (20% TUNEL-positive cells after 24 hours). In the presence of PDGF, a concentration-dependent reduction in programmed cell death could be observed in both the wild-type and TN-C knockout OPC cultures. After 24 hours, at a PDGF concentration of 1 mg/ml, apoptosis in wild-type OPC cultures was halved. In TN-C knockout OPC cultures, apoptosis after 24 hours was also reduced by the action of PDGF, although even at 10 ng/ml, the highest concentration tested, it was still considerably higher (32%) than that observed for the wild-type OPC cultures. After 48 hours PDGF treatment, a protective effect of PDGF could still be observed for wild-type OPCs. However, in the TN-C knockout OPC cultures a complete loss of any protective effects of PDGF was apparent after 48 hours (Garwood *et al.*, 2004).

Hence, in addition to a reduction in the levels of proliferation among the TN-C knockout OPCs in vitro (Garcion *et al.*, 2001), the absence of TN-C appears to contribute to increased levels of programmed cell death in these cells. Furthermore, although PDGF promotes OPC survival, these protective, anti-apoptotic effects are reduced with time of culture for both wild-type and TN-C knockout OPCs. However, in the absence of TN-C, the anti-apoptotic response of TN-C knockout OPCs to the protective effects of PDGF disappears earlier than in the wild-type OPCs. The strong upregulation of TN-C expression in OPCs by the survival factors, CNTF and LIF, further reinforces this interpretation of anti-apoptotic effects of TN-C on this precursor cell population (Garwood *et al.*, 2004).

However, although in vitro a higher level of apoptosis in TN-C knockout OPC cultures was observed, this does not appear to be the case in vivo where reduced levels of apoptosis were found in myelinated tracts of TN-C knockout mice compared to wild-type (Garcion *et al.*, 2001). This discrepancy might be explained by the presence in vivo of factors necessary for the survival of mature oligodendrocytes that are absent in vitro, and it may highlight a compensatory mechanism that serves to limit the effects of reduced OPC proliferation in the mutant.

In TN-C knockout mice, reduced levels of OPC proliferation are observed (Garcion *et al.*, 2001). Given the apparent normality of subsequent myelination in the TN-C knockout, this suggests that there is a mechanism that is correcting for the reduced size of the OPC population in TN-C knockout mice: in normal development, upto 50% of the newly-formed, differentiated, oligodendrocytes die in order to match the final numbers of myelinating oligodendrocytes to their target axons (Barres & Raff, 1999). In TN-C knockout mice, this excess cell population is proportionally smaller and hence requires less pruning. Therefore, the production of a large excess of OPCs relative to the final number of axon-ensheathing oligodendrocytes would appear to be one of the compensatory mechanisms that is operating in order to correct for, and minimise, the otherwise damaging effects of developmental defects. The adaptive capacity of such compensatory mechanisms has been proposed as a key explanation for the relatively benign effects of the TN-C transgenic knockout mice (Steindler *et al.*, 1995; Bartsch, 1996; Jones & Jones, 2000b).

Conclusion

The relatively new field of stem cell biology will continue to be an active area of investigation with ECM components. Specific potential benefits of understanding stem-cell–ECM interactions are prolonged stem-cell survival, proliferation and differentiation in vitro, as well as improved targeting, survival and differentiation in vivo. Neural stem cells reside in niches that regulate their self-renewal, activation and differentiation. Understanding what defines the cellular microenvironment in tissue and especially the niches for stem cells and their progeny, cell precursor populations, is of great relevance to the development of therapeutic strategies that rely on the regeneration of degenerated tissue, whether from transplanted progenitor cells or the manipulation of existing reservoirs of stem cells. Clarifying the role of the ECM in defining and regulating stem cell niches will be a key aspect in the realisation of this potential.

References

Alvarez-Buylla, A., Garcia-Verdugo, J.M. & Tramontin, A.D. (2001) A unified hypothesis on the lineage of neural stem cells. *Nat Rev Neurosci*, **2**, 287-293.

Alvarez-Buylla, A. & Temple, S. (1998) Stem cells in the developing and adult nervous system. *J Neurobiol*, **36**, 105-110.

Barres, B.A. & Raff, M.C. (1999) Axonal control of oligodendrocyte development. *J Cell Biol*, **147**, 1123-1128.

Bartsch, S., Bartsch, U., Dorries, U., Faissner, A., Weller, A., Ekblom, P. & Schachner, M. (1992) Expression of tenascin in the developing and adult cerebellar cortex. *J Neurosci*, **12**, 736-749.

Bartsch, U. (1996) The extracellular matrix molecule tenascin-C: expression in vivo and functional characterization in vitro. *Prog Neurobiol*, **49**, 145-168.

Benoit, B.O., Savarese, T., Joly, M., Engstrom, C.M., Pang, L., Reilly, J., Recht, L.D., Ross, A.H. & Quesenberry, P.J. (2001) Neurotrophin channeling of neural progenitor cell differentiation. *J Neurobiol*, **46**, 265-280.

Blaschuk, K.L., Frost, E.E. & ffrench-Constant, C. (2000) The regulation of proliferation and differentiation in oligodendrocyte progenitor cells by alphaV integrins. *Development*, **127**, 1961-1969.

Bogler, O., Wren, D., Barnett, S.C., Land, H. & Noble, M. (1990) Cooperation between two growth factors promotes extended self-renewal and inhibits differentiation of oligodendrocyte-type-2 astrocyte (O-2A) progenitor cells. *Proc Natl Acad Sci U S A*, **87**, 6368-6372.

Burrows, R.C., Wancio, D., Levitt, P. & Lillien, L. (1997) Response diversity and the timing of progenitor cell maturation are regulated by developmental changes in EGFR expression in the cortex. *Neuron*, **19**, 251-267.

Carey, D.J. (1997) Syndecans: multifunctional cell-surface co-receptors. *Biochem J*, **327**, 1-16.

Casaccia-Bonnefil, P. (2000) Cell death in the oligodendrocyte lineage: a molecular perspective of life/death decisions in development and disease. *Glia*, **29**, 124-135.

Chiquet-Ehrismann, R. & Chiquet, M. (2003) Tenascins: regulation and putative functions during pathological stress. *J Pathol*, **200**, 488-499.

Chothia, C. & Jones, E.Y. (1997) The molecular structure of cell adhesion molecules. *Annu Rev Biochem*, **66**, 823-862.

Ciccolini, F. & Svendsen, C.N. (1998) Fibroblast growth factor 2 (FGF-2) promotes acquisition of epidermal growth factor (EGF) responsiveness in mouse striatal precursor cells: identification of neural precursors responding to both EGF and FGF-2. *J Neurosci*, **18**, 7869-7880.

Colognato, H., Baron, W., Avellana-Adalid, V., Relvas, J.B., Baron-Van Evercooren, A., Georges-Labouesse, E. & ffrench-Constant, C. (2002) CNS integrins switch growth factor signalling to promote target-dependent survival. *Nat Cell Biol*, **4**, 833-841.

Crossin, K.L. (1996) Tenascin: a multifunctional extracellular matrix protein with a restricted distribution in development and disease. *J Cell Biochem*, **61**, 592-598.

Cukierman, E., Pankov, R. & Yamada, K.M. (2002) Cell interactions with three-dimensional matrices. *Curr Opin Cell Biol*, **14**, 633-639.

Czyz, J. & Wobus, A. (2001) Embryonic stem cell differentiation: the role of extracellular factors. *Differentiation*, **68**, 167-174.

Deller, T., Haas, C.A., Naumann, T., Joester, A., Faissner, A. & Frotscher, M. (1997) Up-regulation of astrocyte-derived tenascin-C correlates with neurite outgrowth in the rat dentate gyrus after unilateral entorhinal cortex lesion. *Neuroscience*, **81**, 829-846.

Doetsch, F. (2003) A niche for adult neural stem cells. *Curr Opin Genet Dev*, **13**, 543-550.

Doetsch, F., Garcia-Verdugo, J.M. & Alvarez-Buylla, A. (1997) Cellular composition and three-dimensional organization of the subventricular germinal zone in the adult mammalian brain. *J Neurosci*, **17**, 5046-5061.

Faissner, A. (1997) The tenascin gene family in axon growth and guidance. *Cell Tissue Res*, **290**, 331-341.

Faissner, A. & Kruse, J. (1990) J1/tenascin is a repulsive substrate for central nervous system neurons. *Neuron*, **5**, 627-637.

Faissner, A. & Steindler, D. (1995) Boundaries and inhibitory molecules in developing neural tissues. *Glia*, **13**, 233-254.

Frost, E., Kiernan, B.W., Faissner, A. & ffrench-Constant, C. (1996) Regulation of oligodendrocyte precursor migration by extracellular matrix: evidence for substrate-specific inhibition of migration by tenascin-C. *Dev Neurosci*, **18**, 266-273.

Frost, E.E., Buttery, P.C., Milner, R. & ffrench-Constant, C. (1999) Integrins mediate a neuronal survival signal for oligodendrocytes. *Curr Biol*, **9**, 1251-1254.

Garcion, E., Faissner, A. & ffrench-Constant, C. (2001) Knockout mice reveal a contribution of the extracellular matrix molecule tenascin-C to neural precursor proliferation and migration. *Development*, **128**, 2485-2496.

Garcion, E., Halilagic, A., Faissner, A. & ffrench-Constant, C. (2004) Generation of an environmental niche for neural stem cell development by the extracellular matrix molecule tenascin-C. *Development*, **131**, 3423-3432.

Garwood, J., Garcion, E., Dobbertin, A., Heck, N., Calco, V., ffrench-Constant, C. & Faissner, A. (2004) The extracellular matrix glycoprotein Tenascin-C is expressed by oligodendrocyte precursor cells and required for the regulation of maturation rate, survival and responsiveness to platelet-derived growth factor. *Eur J Neurosci*, **20**, 2524-2540.

Garwood, J., Heck, N., Rigato, F. & Faissner, A. (2002) The extracellular matrix in neural development, plasticity and regeneration. In Walz, W. (ed.) *The neuronal microenvironment*. Humana Press, Totowa, New Jersey, USA, pp. 109-158.

Garwood, J., Rigato, F., Heck, N. & Faissner, A. (2001) Tenascin glycoproteins and the complementary ligand DSD-1-PG/phosphacan – structuring the neural extracellular matrix during development and repair. *Restor Neurol Neurosci*, **19**, 51-64.

Garwood, J., Schnadelbach, O., Clement, A., Schutte, K., Bach, A. & Faissner, A. (1999) DSD-1-proteoglycan is the mouse homolog of phosphacan and displays opposing effects on neurite outgrowth dependent on neuronal lineage. *J Neurosci*, **19**, 3888-3899.

Gates, M.A., Thomas, L.B., Howard, E.M., Laywell, E.D., Sajin, B., Faissner, A., Gotz, B., Silver, J. & Steindler, D.A. (1995) Cell and molecular analysis of the developing and adult mouse subventricular zone of the cerebral hemispheres. *J Comp Neurol*, **361**, 249-266.

Gotz, B., Scholze, A., Clement, A., Joester, A., Schutte, K., Wigger, F., Frank, R., Spiess, E., Ekblom, P. & Faissner, A. (1996) Tenascin-C contains distinct adhesive, anti-adhesive, and neurite outgrowth promoting sites for neurons. *J Cell Biol*, **132**, 681-699.

Gotz, M., Bolz, J., Joester, A. & Faissner, A. (1997) Tenascin-C synthesis and influence on axonal growth during rat cortical development. *Eur J Neurosci*, **9**, 496-506.

Gotz, M., Stoykova, A. & Gruss, P. (1998) Pax6 controls radial glia differentiation in the cerebral cortex. *Neuron*, **21**, 1031-1044.

Gross, R.E., Mehler, M.F., Mabie, P.C., Zang, Z., Santschi, L. & Kessler, J.A. (1996) Bone morphogenetic proteins promote astroglial lineage commitment by mammalian subventricular zone progenitor cells. *Neuron*, **17**, 595-606.

Gumbiner, B.M. (1996) Cell adhesion: the molecular basis of tissue architecture and morphogenesis. *Cell*, **84**, 345-357.

Gustafsson, E. & Fassler, R. (2000) Insights into extracellular matrix functions from mutant mouse models. *Exp Cell Res*, **261**, 52-68.

Hartfuss, E., Galli, R., Heins, N. & Gotz, M. (2001) Characterization of CNS precursor subtypes and radial glia. *Dev Biol*, **229**, 15-30.

Heck, N., Garwood, J., Loeffler, J.P., Larmet, Y. & Faissner, A. (2004) Differential upregulation of extracellular matrix molecules associated with the appearance of granule cell dispersion and mossy fiber sprouting during epileptogenesis in a murine model of temporal lobe epilepsy. *Neuroscience*, **129**, 309-324.

Hubbard, S.R. (1999) Structural analysis of receptor tyrosine kinases. *Prog Biophys Mol Biol*, **71**, 343-358.

Husmann, K., Faissner, A. & Schachner, M. (1992) Tenascin promotes cerebellar granule cell migration and neurite outgrowth by different domains in the fibronectin type III repeats. *J Cell Biol*, **116**, 1475-1486.

Jankovski, A. & Sotelo, C. (1996) Subventricular zone-olfactory bulb migratory pathway in the adult mouse: cellular composition and specificity as determined by heterochronic and heterotopic transplantation. *J Comp Neurol*, **371**, 376-396.

Joester, A. & Faissner, A. (1999) Evidence for combinatorial variability of tenascin-C isoforms and developmental regulation in the mouse central nervous system. *J Biol Chem*, **274**, 17144-17151.

Joester, A. & Faissner, A. (2001) The structure and function of tenascins in the nervous system. *Matrix Biol*, **20**, 13-22.

Johe, K.K., Hazel, T.G., Muller, T., Dugich-Djordjevic, M.M. & McKay, R.D. (1996) Single factors direct the differentiation of stem cells from the fetal and adult central nervous system. *Genes Dev*, **10**, 3129-3140.

Jones, F.S. & Jones, P.L. (2000a) The tenascin family of ECM glycoproteins: structure, function, and regulation during embryonic development and tissue remodeling. *Dev Dyn*, **218**, 235-259.

Jones, P.L. & Jones, F.S. (2000b) Tenascin-C in development and disease: gene regulation and cell function. *Matrix Biol*, **19**, 581-596.

Julliard, A.K. & Hartmann, D.J. (1998) Spatiotemporal patterns of expression of extracellular matrix molecules in the developing and adult rat olfactory system. *Neuroscience*, **84**, 1135-1150.

Kiernan, B.W., Gotz, B., Faissner, A. & ffrench-Constant, C. (1996) Tenascin-C inhibits oligodendrocyte precursor cell migration by both adhesion-dependent and adhesion-independent mechanisms. *Mol Cell Neurosci*, **7**, 322-335.

Kilpatrick, T.J. & Bartlett, P.F. (1995) Cloned multipotential precursors from the mouse cerebrum require FGF-2, whereas glial restricted precursors are stimulated with either FGF-2 or EGF. *J Neurosci*, **15**, 3653-3661.

Kleinman, H.K., Philp, D. & Hoffman, M.P. (2003) Role of the extracellular matrix in morphogenesis. *Curr Opin Biotechnol*, **14**, 526-532.

Kusakabe, M., Mangiarini, L., Laywell, E.D., Bates, G.P., Yoshiki, A., Hiraiwa, N., Inoue, J. & Steindler, D.A. (2001) Loss of cortical and thalamic neuronal tenascin-C expression in a transgenic mouse expressing exon 1 of the human Huntington disease gene. *J Comp Neurol*, **430**, 485-500.

Levison, S.W., Chuang, C., Abramson, B.J. & Goldman, J.E. (1993) The migrational patterns and developmental fates of glial precursors in the rat subventricular zone are temporally regulated. *Development*, **119**, 611-622.

Li, S., Harrison, D., Carbonetto, S., Fassler, R., Smyth, N., Edgar, D. & Yurchenco, P.D. (2002) Matrix assembly, regulation, and survival functions of laminin and its receptors in embryonic stem cell differentiation. *J Cell Biol*, **157**, 1279-1290.

Lillien, L. & Raphael, H. (2000) BMP and FGF regulate the development of EGF-responsive neural progenitor cells. *Development*, **127**, 4993-5005.

Lim, D.A., Tramontin, A.D., Trevejo, J.M., Herrera, D.G., Garcia-Verdugo, J.M. & Alvarez-Buylla, A. (2000) Noggin antagonizes BMP signaling to create a niche for adult neurogenesis. *Neuron*, **28**, 713-726.

Lochter, A., Vaughan, L., Kaplony, A., Prochiantz, A., Schachner, M. & Faissner, A. (1991) J1/tenascin in substrate-bound and soluble form displays contrary effects on neurite outgrowth. *J Cell Biol*, **113**, 1159-1171.

Meiners, S., Powell, E.M. & Geller, H.M. (1995) A distinct subset of tenascin/CS-6-PG-rich astrocytes restricts neuronal growth in vitro. *J Neurosci*, **15**, 8096-8108.

Milev, P., Fischer, D., Haring, M., Schulthess, T., Margolis, R.K., Chiquet-Ehrismann, R. & Margolis, R.U. (1997) The fibrinogen-like globe of tenascin-C mediates its interactions with neurocan and phosphacan/protein-tyrosine phosphatase-zeta/beta. *J Biol Chem*, **272**, 15501-15509.

Miller, R.H. (2002) Regulation of oligodendrocyte development in the vertebrate CNS. *Prog Neurobiol*, **67**, 451-467.

Miragall, F., Kadmon, G., Faissner, A., Antonicek, H. & Schachner, M. (1990) Retention of J1/tenascin and the polysialylated form of the neural cell adhesion molecule (N-CAM) in the adult olfactory bulb. *J Neurocytol*, **19**, 899-914.

Nishio, T., Kawaguchi, S., Iseda, T., Kawasaki, T. & Hase, T. (2003) Secretion of tenascin-C by cultured astrocytes: regulation of cell proliferation and process elongation. *Brain Res*, **990**, 129-140.

O'Brien, T.F., Faissner, A., Schachner, M. & Steindler, D.A. (1992) Afferent-boundary interactions in the developing neostriatal mosaic. *Brain Res Dev Brain Res*, **65**, 259-267.

Ohta, M., Sakai, T., Saga, Y., Aizawa, S. & Saito, M. (1998) Suppression of hematopoietic activity in tenascin-C-deficient mice. *Blood*, **91**, 4074-4083.

Ono, K., Bansal, R., Payne, J., Rutishauser, U. & Miller, R.H. (1995) Early development and dispersal of oligodendrocyte precursors in the embryonic chick spinal cord. *Development*, **121**, 1743-1754.

Panchision, D.M., Pickel, J.M., Studer, L., Lee, S.H., Turner, P.A., Hazel, T.G. & McKay, R.D. (2001) Sequential actions of BMP receptors control neural precursor cell production and fate. *Genes Dev*, **15**, 2094-2110.

Pearlman, A.L. & Sheppard, A.M. (1996) Extracellular matrix in early cortical development. *Prog Brain Res*, **108**, 117-134.

Peles, E., Schlessinger, J. & Grumet, M. (1998) Multi-ligand interactions with receptor-like protein tyrosine phosphatase beta: implications for intercellular signaling. *Trends Biochem Sci*, **23**, 121-124.

Qian, X., Shen, Q., Goderie, S.K., He, W., Capela, A., Davis, A.A. & Temple, S. (2000) Timing of CNS cell generation: a programmed sequence of neuron and glial cell production from isolated murine cortical stem cells. *Neuron*, **28**, 69-80.

Raff, M.C., Miller, R.H. & Noble, M. (1983) A glial progenitor cell that develops in vitro into an astrocyte or an oligodendrocyte depending on culture medium. *Nature*, **303**, 390-396.

Ramalho-Santos, M., Yoon, S., Matsuzaki, Y., Mulligan, R.C. & Melton, D.A. (2002) "Stemness": transcriptional profiling of embryonic and adult stem cells. *Science*, **298**, 597-600.

Rigato, F., Garwood, J., Calco, V., Heck, N., Faivre-Sarrailh, C. & Faissner, A. (2002) Tenascin-C promotes neurite outgrowth of embryonic hippocampal neurons through the alternatively spliced fibronectin type III BD domains via activation of the cell adhesion molecule F3/contactin. *J Neurosci*, **22**, 6596-6609.

Ruoslahti, E. (1996) Integrin signaling and matrix assembly. *Tumour Biol*, **17**, 117-124.

Schenk, S., Hintermann, E., Bilban, M., Koshikawa, N., Hojilla, C., Khokha, R. & Quaranta, V. (2003) Binding to EGF receptor of a laminin-5 EGF-like fragment liberated during MMP-dependent mammary gland involution. *J Cell Biol*, **161**, 197-209.

Spradling, A., Drummond-Barbosa, D. & Kai, T. (2001) Stem cells find their niche. *Nature*, **414**, 98-104.

Steindler, D.A., Settles, D., Erickson, H.P., Laywell, E.D., Yoshiki, A., Faissner, A. & Kusakabe, M. (1995) Tenascin knockout mice: barrels, boundary molecules, and glial scars. *J Neurosci*, **15**, 1971-1983.

Streuli, C. (1999) Extracellular matrix remodelling and cellular differentiation. *Curr Opin Cell Biol*, **11**, 634-640.

Sudhakar, A., Sugimoto, H., Yang, C., Lively, J., Zeisberg, M. & Kalluri, R. (2003) Human tumstatin and human endostatin exhibit distinct antiangiogenic activities mediated by alpha v beta 3 and alpha 5 beta 1 integrins. *Proc Natl Acad Sci U S A*, **100**, 4766-4771.

Tang, D.G., Tokumoto, Y.M. & Raff, M.C. (2000) Long-term culture of purified postnatal oligodendrocyte precursor cells. Evidence for an intrinsic maturation program that plays out over months. *J Cell Biol*, **148**, 971-984.

Taylor, J., Pesheva, P. & Schachner, M. (1993) Influence of janusin and tenascin on growth cone behavior in vitro. *J Neurosci Res*, **35**, 347-362.

Temple, S. (2001) The development of neural stem cells. *Nature*, **414**, 112-117.

Trapp, B.D., Nishiyama, A., Cheng, D. & Macklin, W. (1997) Differentiation and death of premyelinating oligodendrocytes in developing rodent brain. *J Cell Biol*, **137**, 459-468.

Vos, J.P., Gard, A.L. & Pfeiffer, S.E. (1996) Regulation of oligodendrocyte cell survival and differentiation by ciliary neurotrophic factor, leukemia inhibitory factor, oncostatin M, and interleukin-6. *Perspect Dev Neurobiol*, **4**, 39-52.

Zhang, Z.Y. (1998) Protein-tyrosine phosphatases: biological function, structural characteristics, and mechanism of catalysis. *Crit Rev Biochem Mol Biol*, **33**, 1-52.

In: Neural Stem Cell Research
Editor: Eric V. Grier, pp. 51-75

ISBN: 1-59454-846-3
© 2006 Nova Science Publishers, Inc.

Chapter 3

TOWARDS A MOLECULAR SIGNATURE OF NEURAL STEM CELLS

Martin H. Maurer[*] and Wolfgang Kuschinsky

Dept. of Physiology and Pathophysiology, University of Heidelberg, Im Neuenheimer
Feld 326, 69120 Heidelberg, Germany

Abstract

Neural stem cells can be isolated from various regions of the adult brain, including the regions with spontaneous neurogenesis, i. e. the dentate gyrus of the hippocampus, and the subventricular zone. With regard to proliferation and differentiation, the properties of these adult neural stem and progenitor cells have been defined as (i) postnatal cells in the adult brain capable of cell division, (ii) self-renewing the stem cell precursor pool, and (iii) giving rise to differentiated cells of the neural, astrocytic, and oligodendrocytic lineage. Whereas their proliferative activity and differentiation potential has been well characterized, a generally accepted cellular marker for the neural stem and progenitor cell has not yet been established. In this article, efforts are described to specify such markers.

Most of the promising candidates for neural stem cell markers such as nestin, doublecortin, Musashi-1, or Mcm2, are not exclusively expressed in neural stem cells, or when expressed, this happens only during a short time period of development. Consequently, the search for specific markers has been expanded to new high-throughput techniques based on genomic, transcriptomic, or proteomic screening of embryonic and adult neural stem cells.

In this chapter, we discuss the use of the most prominent presumptive neural stem cell markers currently in use to identify these cells. We evaluate their expression with regard to time and specificity, and summarize the current standard protocols for neural stem cell staining. In the second section of this chapter, we compare gene expression patterns of neural stem cells, which exist on the genome or transcriptome level, with gene

---

[*] Corresponding author: Dr. Martin H. Maurer, Dept. of Physiology and Pathophysiology, University of Heidelberg, Im Neuenheimer Feld 326, 69120 Heidelberg. Phone: +49-6221-54-4075, Fax. +49-6221-54-4561, Email: maurer@uni-hd.de

expression patterns of other stem cells. In the third section of the chapter, we review the current literature on stem cell proteomics. Protein inventories of neural stem cells at different times of development and different status of differentiation have been created as a basis of protein expression analysis. Now, these inventories are increasingly used for differential protein expression studies.

We summarize the pros and cons of the current stem cell markers and comment on large-scale genomic, transcriptomic, and proteomic approaches for the search of a stem cell specific expression pattern. We conclude that agreement on the cellular markers of neural stem cells is still lacking.

Introduction

The fundamental aspects of cell biology have been established in the cell theory of Matthias Schleiden and Theodor Schwann in the middle of the 19th century who described the morphology and function of the plant and animal cell [1]. Together with Rudolf Virchow's concept of cellular inheritance ("omnis cellula e cellula", all cells are derived from another cell) [2] and the morphological advances in microscopy made by Camillo Golgi [3] and Santiago Ramón y Cajal [4] on the dawn of the 20th century, these works constitutes the backbone of modern cell physiology. In this concept, stem cells play an essential role in the generation and regeneration of specific cells, tissues, and organs. The formation of these, as well as their interaction in the complete organism, is a highly regulated process controlled by developmental programs which are determined genetically and controlled by the microenvironment [5-8]. From the earliest stem cell, the zygote, all other cells are derived by continuous cell divisions. After differentiation, the newly formed cells are apparently distinct from the cell or their origin, both with respect to morphology and function, but stem cells have been found to reside in all tissues investigated so far throughout the life of an individual. This is highly obvious in fast proliferating organs such as skin, liver, bone marrow and intestine epithelia, but stem cells are rare in slowly renewing tissues such as the brain.

During development, stem cells can be classified hierarchically by their potentiality, i. e. the extent to which they are able to produce functionally differentiated progeny [9-11] (Fig. 1). Starting from the totipotent zygote, which gives rise to all sorts of cells which constitute the intact organism, pluripotent embryonic stem cells evolve. The pluripotent embryonic stem cell cannot form the complete organism any more, but it can differentiate into any kind of cell. A more restricted kind of stem cell, the multipotent stem cell develops from the embryonic stem cell. It is also the type of stem cell which persists in the adult organism. Multipotent stem cells are able to differentiate into all cell types of the same germinal layer. During differentiation, they produce progenitor cells of the respective tissue. Progenitor cells are restricted to specific functional cell lineages of the organ they reside in. They are yet not fully functional cells, but they give rise to the terminally differentiated cell type which fulfills the functional requirements of the respective tissue [12-16].

As to the brain, Santiago Ramón y Cajal's central dogma of neurobiology has stated that no regeneration shall occur in the brain after embryonic and fetal development. His dogma has been invalidated within the last 10-15 years by the finding that multipotent stem cells also

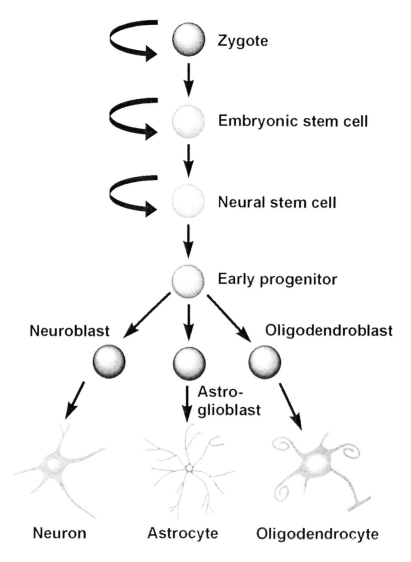

Fig. 1. The classical developmental view of a hierarchical system in stem cell biology. The totipotent zygote gives rise to the pluripotent embryonic stem cell, which develops to the multipotent neural stem cell retaining the ability for self-renewal. This ability is lost in the later stages of the unrestricted early progenitors, the lineage-restricted precursor cells (neuroblasts, astroglioblasts, oligodendroblast), and the terminally differentiated brain cells, i. e. neurons, astrocytes, and oligodendrocytes.

reside in the mature brain. These brain-derived stem cells have been isolated from various regions of the brain not only during development, but also in adulthood. The highest densities of neural stem cells can be found in the dentate gyrus of the hippocampus [17-21], and the subventricular zone [22-24]. Moreover, stem cells have been isolated from the cerebral cortex [25-27], the ventricular zone [28], the substantia nigra [29], and both the subependymal [30] and the ependymal layer [31, 32]. In distinct brain areas, other cell types such as astrocytes [24, 33, 34] or radial glia [35-38] seem to have stem cell properties.

The interest in neural stem cells is steadily increasing (Fig. 2). After some of the most important factors influencing survival, migration, and maturation had been understood [39, 40], their therapeutical potential to replace diseased brain tissue became apparent. Whereas adult hematopoietic stem cells had made their way into the clinical setting already some 20-30 years ago, the use of neural stem cells is still limited to experimental studies. Although promising results in the fields of cerebrovascular diseases such as stroke, neurodegenerative diseases such as Parkinson's or Alzheimer's disease, or traumata of the spinal cord have been reported, no standard therapies using neural stem cells have yet been established [41-44].

What are the unique properties of neural stem cells? Similar to other stem cells, brain-derived neural stem cells have the ability to proliferate, i. e. to divide into daughter cells thus increasing the pool of self-renewing neural stem cells. Besides the proliferation aspects, also differentiation processes have been used to define neural stem cells. These cells must give rise to at least one of the three cellular lineages in the brain, neurons, astrocytes, and oligodendrocytes. Currently, it is controversial whether a unique progenitor cell type exists *in vivo* which has the potential to give rise to all three lineages (trilineage potential), or whether different progenitor cell lines give rise to either lineage. Besides the morphological prerequisites, the terminally differentiated cells derived from neural stem cells must provide the typical functional properties of the residing cells. For example, when they differentiate into neurons, the cells must be electrophysiologically active and be able to integrate into neuronal circuits [45, 46]. When they differentiate into oligodendrocytes, they must sheath axons, and astrocytes must regulate cell communication. Additionally, stem cells isolated from the nervous system are not unique to produce cells of brain cell phenotypes. This can also be done by stem cells isolated from other organs, like bone marrow [47-51], umbilical cord blood [49, 52], and several other organs [53].

In most studies, the identity of differentiated cells has been verified by the expression of "marker proteins" for neurons, astrocytes, and oligodendrocytes ([53], Appendix E.i. "How Do Researchers Use Markers to Identify Stem Cells?"). Besides the problems of the specificity of these markers which are expressed even in the differentiated cells, consensus does not exist as to specific markers of their progenitors [54-56]. Therefore, in the absence of reliable markers, functional definitions of neural stem cells have been proposed [13, 15, 57]. The least common denominator states that neural stem cells must be capable of proliferating and self-renewing as well as giving rise to at least one lineage of brain-derived cells, may it be neurons, astrocytes, or oligodendrocytes (Of note, not necessarily all three of them may be formed, thus the three-lineage progeny is still a postulate [58, 59]).

One possibility to obtain high numbers of neural stem/progenitor cells is to expand the cells in the neurosphere assay [60-63]. In this assay, single cells isolated from specific brain regions grow in large free-floating cell clusters resulting in hundreds or even thousands of neural stem/progenitor cells contained in one neurosphere. Although this number is not exactly defined, the neurosphere assay still constitutes an important assay to study neural stem cell function.

In this chapter, we will discuss the experimental basis of the search for neural stem cell markers, followed by recent alternative concepts of neural stem cell definitions based on integrative systems biology. Special emphasis will be given to stem cell proteomics.

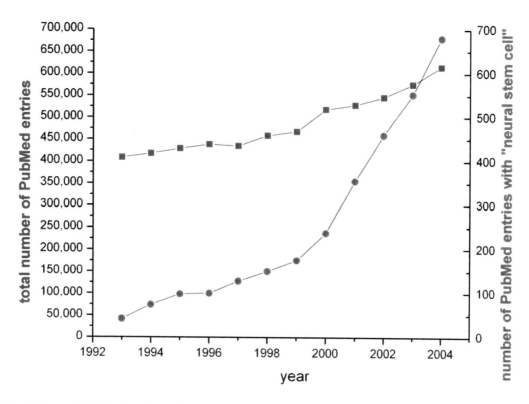

Fig. 2. Since the isolation of neural stem cells from the adult brain, the term "neural stem cell" saw a tremendous increase in its number of PubMed entries. Whereas there was a steady increase of about 3-5% in the total number of PubMed entries (blue squares), the number of publications using the term "neural stem cell" (and its derivations) in any PubMed search field grew exponentially (red dots). In 2004, it occurred in almost 680 publications, representing about 0.11% of all PubMed entries.

Neural Stem Cell Markers

The current definition of neural stem cells by their properties of self-renewal and multipotency [13] is clearly functional, compared to other stem cell definitions such as that of hematopoietic stem cells. For hematopoietic stem cells, the expression of a combination of specific cellular surface markers has been established as typical [64-66]. Unfortunately, no such definition has been found for neural stem cells [54, 67, 15]. Although several presumptive markers have been proposed (reviewed in [68]), none of them comprehends all subtypes of neural stem cells at any given point of time or region in development (Figs 3, 4). In all cases, the candidate marker is only expressed in a certain subfraction of neural stem cells. The National Institutes of Health of the U.S.A. list on their website an overview over the most discussed markers [53] (http://stemcells.nih.gov/info/scireport).

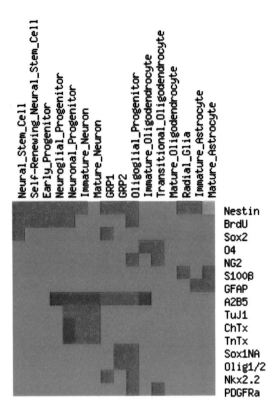

Fig. 3. Expression of "specific" antigens in neural stem cells and differentiated progeny. The overlap in the expression pattern (red box) does not allow an unequivocal identification of neural stem cells (data from [73] and [80]). (green box: expression is unclear).

The most prominent of these markers is the intermediate filament protein nestin [69]. Nestin is expressed in the cellular population identified as neural stem cell [70]. However, it is also expressed in embryonic precursors of the neuroectodermal, entodermal, and mesodermal lineage. This precludes the use of nestin as an exclusive marker of neural stem cells. Apparently, nestin is expressed in proliferating neural tissue during development and in regenerative tissue during later stages which includes its expression in the adult. Although the expression of nestin is not exclusive for neural stem cells, its expression is characteristic for precursor cells of multi-lineage potential [71]. Recently, also electrophysiologically different subpopulations of nestin-positive cells have been identified [72], supporting the hypothesis of the existence of several heterogeneous neural stem cell populations in the brain. Moreover, nestin-immunoreactivity is lost in the oligodendrocytic and astrocytic precursors [73].

Indirect evidence for the existence of neural stem cells can be obtained from labeling dividing cells, for example with the thymidine analog 5-bromo-2-deoxyuridine (BrdU) which is incorporated into the replicated DNA during mitosis [74]. It has to be kept in mind that BrdU will label all proliferating cells despite of their various histological origin. Therefore, endothelial and microglial cells will also be labeled. Additionally, during repeated cell

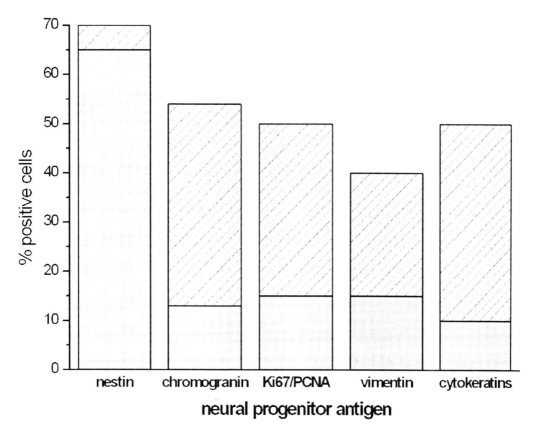

Fig. 4. Example of quantitative assessment of "markers" expressed in neural stem cells. The columns show the fraction of immunopositive neural stem cells in relation to all neural stem cells counted. The filled part shows the minimum number, hatched part the maximum number of cells obtained from different investigations. The extensive variation is mainly depending on the stem cell preparation, age of the donor, developmental stage, and region of origin (data from [174]).

divisions, BrdU applied at one time point becomes more and more diluted [75], resulting in a lower count for BrdU-positive cells than actually replicating. Another potential problem of BrdU is that slow-dividing cells, or cells resting from the cell cycle, may not be labeled by a single dose of BrdU. Typically, neural stem cell populations of only slow cellular turnover will not be labeled by BrdU [76]. Therefore, BrdU, like the proliferating cell marker Ki67, can be used as cell cycle marker for proliferative cells in general. However, these markers also do not label all *stem* cells, but only the proliferating ones [77]. With regard to slow-cycling neural stem cell populations, the replication factor Mcm2 has been proposed which is expressed in the G1 phase [78], but only the Musashi1 protein co-localized with Mcm2 unequivocally, whereas the expression of other proposed markers such as nestin differs from Mcm2 expression. In conclusion, it seems that also Mcm2 labels only a subfraction of neural stem cells.

The expression of markers for mature brain cells may be taken as criterion to exclude the presence of precursor cells. This definition *ex contrario* would exclude all cells as neural stem cells expressing, e. g., the Microtubule-associated protein-2 (MAP-2), neural tubulin ß$_{III}$, neurofilament proteins (NF), synaptophysin, or the neuron-specific tau (τ) protein as well as the Myelin basic protein (MPB), and the O1 protein which are both found in mature oligodendrocytes.

Another problem arises from the missing specificity of a marker which has been considered to be specific for astrocytes in the past, i. e. the Glial Fibrillary Acidic Protein (GFAP). The fact that GFAP has also been found in neural stem cells [24] has raised the question about the identity both of glial cells and neural stem cells [79, 15, 34, 80]. Currently, it seems that certain neural stem cells can express GFAP, but this does not hold for all of them; on the other hand, certain GFAP-positive cells can be regarded as neural stem cells, but again not all of them. Especially the GFAP-positive radial glia cells [81, 82] turned out not only to direct neuronal precursor migration towards the cerebral cortex, but also to generate new neurons themselves [83, 84]. Therefore, care must be taken when considering GFAP as an astrocytic marker. Although GFAP is not exclusively expressed in astrocytes, but also in ependymal cells and tanycytes [85, 35, 86], it is still used a astrocytic marker. Instead of showing the existence of astrocytes, the expression of GFAP may indicate the potency of cells to function as stem cells, since astrocytes serve both as stem cell reservoir and maintain the germinal stem cell niche [87].

To illustrate the heterogeneity of cells of neuronal origin, we will discuss the example of radial glia cells further. Radial glia cells span processes from the ventricle to the brain surface. Newborn neurons migrate along these processes towards their final position [88]. This concept of a purely guiding function of radial glia has changed in recent years when evidence arose that radial glia cells can act as neural progenitors themselves [37, 38]. On the other hand, regional differences in the fate of cells derived from radial glia exist in the brain: for example, radial glia cells give rise to most cortical projection neurons but only to few neurons in the basal ganglia [38]. These findings support the idea of regional subpopulations of neural stem cells specified by local environmental factors. One of the factors regulating radial glial cell fate in development is the transcription factor Pax6 [89]. In adult neurogenesis, Pax6 regulates the differentiation of interneurons in the olfactory bulb [90]. Therefore, Pax6 is involved in the regionalization of neural stem cells, also in combination with a second transcription factor Olig2 [90]. Of note, Pax6 is not exclusively expressed in neural stem cells, but also in enteroendocrine cells and photoreceptors [91, 92].

The RNA-binding proteins Musashi1 (Msi1) and Musashi2 (Msi2) are also not specific for neural stem cells. They label proliferating embryonic pluripotent neural precursors as well as adult neural stem cells [93-96], but also other neuroepithelial and mesenchymal cells.

Markers which are expressed only by subsets of neural stem cells include doublecortin (DCX), a protein associated with microtubules and involved in cellular dynamics [97]. Doublecortin is found in migrating neural stem cells in development and indicates active zones of neurogenesis in the adult [98, 99]. Other presumptive markers include members of the SOX transcription factor family [100], members of developmental signaling pathways such as Sonic Hedgehog (SHH), transcription factors of the Pax and Hox gene families, Noggin and the transmembrane receptor Notch [70], as well as the cell-surface protein CD133 (Prominin-1) [101]. Unfortunately, none of these proteins seems to be specific for neural stem cells in the sense that there is an exclusive expression only in neural stem cells and in all (sub-)types of neural stem cells.

Genomic and Transcriptomic Screening

The terms genomics and transcriptomics describe two disciplines which allow to analyze the whole genome, or the complete set of transcripts thereof, respectively. This is yet an idealistic view because of the large number of transcripts to be described, but with an increasing number of organisms of which whole genomic sequences are available, the number of genes or transcripts which can be analyzed simultaneously is steadily increasing.

To this end, a large number of methods has been developed for genomic or transcriptomic expression analysis. High-throughput screening methods for gene/transcript expression include microarrays, Differential Display, DD; Restriction-Mediated Differential Display, RMDD; Amplified Fragment Length Polymorphism, AFLP), tag sequencing (e. g. Massively Parallel Signature Sequencing, MPSS; Serial Analysis of Gene Expression, SAGE), and subtractive/competitive hybridization techniques (e. g. Suppression Subtractive Hybridization, SHH) (reviewed in [102]).

Whereas all of these methods are highly useful in specific applications, microarray studies are more frequently used, also with regard to expression analysis in neural stem cells. Moreover, efforts are made to standardize microarray experiments [103], which makes it easier to compare different experiments. In a typical microarray experiment, the sample RNA species are extracted from cells, tissues, or organs, respectively. The RNA is reversely transcribed into cDNA by random priming or only mRNA is transcribed using oligo(dT) primers. It is possible to incorporate fluorescent dyes in the nascent cDNA strand, or the cDNA is labeled after transcription. Then, the sample cDNA is hybridized to immobilized complementary probe sequences on the microarray surface [104-107].

Dual labeling of two samples allows the direct competitive hybridization of the two samples on the same microarray. After scanning the fluorescent intensities of both fluorophores, the ratios of the signals can be used to relatively quantify the number of transcripts [108, 109, 107]. The differentially expressed sequences can be compared by bioinformatic tools to identify target sequences and interaction partners on the DNA or RNA levels [110-112] as well as to analyze gene expression pathways [113-116].

Microarray studies are an integrative tool in developmental biology for studying "functional genomics" [117-120]. They have supplemented data obtained from other sources such as in situ hybridization, or phenotyping of transgenic mice. The application of microarrays to neural stem cells has been enlarged in parallel to the improvement of cell culture techniques. Large numbers of neural stem cells can now be cultured and isolated which allows to extract an amount of DNA or RNA sufficient for microarray experiments. Several studies have described the changes which occur in the transcriptome of neural stem cells during differentiation. These dramatic changes in morphology and function during differentiation are correlated with significant changes in gene expression.

Using microarray technology, five stages of neural stem cell differentiation have been identified based on characteristic patterns of gene expression [121, 122]. Starting from the proliferating, immature cell, the molecular processes underlying mitosis are down-regulated. The cells then exit the cell cycle. Typical genes involved in this stage encode for cyclins, for replicating enzymes such as DNA polymerase, and for transcription factors. The second and third stages are dedicated to the establishment of functional signaling cascades. The cells start to communicate with each other as well as with the extracellular matrix. They spread processes and establish cell-cell contacts by regulating the expression of cell adhesion molecules, extracellular matrix proteins, and cytoskeletal proteins. Moreover, the cell-cell contacts are enlarged to form first synaptic contacts, and neurotransmitters are synthesized. In the fourth stage, the differentiating cells start to detach from the surface or from neighboring cells and begin to migrate. This requires the expression of specific metabolic components and of cytoskeletal proteins. In the final stage, cells mature and differentiate terminally, which correlates with the expression of proteins specific for neurons or glial cells.

In several microarray studies neural stem cells have been propagated in culture for extended periods of time [123-125]. No major changes in gene expression occurred in the cycling undifferentiated cells over time, some of which have been kept in culture for more than six years. When differentiation was initiated by specific *in vitro* differentiation protocols, the long-term cultured cells had maintained their ability to differentiate into neurons and glial cells. No difference was found to freshly-prepared or short-term cultured neural stem cells. During differentiation, genes were differentially expressed encoding for regulatory pathways activated in cell cycle, growth and proliferation, apoptosis, migration, axon guidance, synaptogenesis, cell morphology, interaction with the extracellular matrix, and neurotransmitter synthesis.

Changes in the expression of genes during differentiation were not exclusively confined to genes involved directly in cell proliferation and differentiation. Differential expression of genes and transcripts in neural stem cells under differentiating conditions also occurred in developmental signaling pathways [7, 8]. These developmental pathways are responsible for pattern formation in the central nervous system defining the spatial orientation of the neuraxis (dorsal-ventral, caudal-rostral, medial-lateral), the guidance of the migrating neural stem cells, as well as the control of cell number and cell fate with respect to asymmetric division [126-129].

Some of these molecular signaling pathways activated during differentiation encompass Sonic Hedgehog (Shh), Notch, TGF-beta, and Wnt signaling as well as transcription factors from the Paired Box (Pax) and Homeobox (Hox) families [70, 130]. Of note, in most microarray studies investigating gene expression in differentiating neural stem cells, at least one member of these signaling pathways has been identified, which can either be the cell surface receptor, intracellular effectors, or nuclear target sequences.

The term "stemness" summarizes the attributes and properties of neural stem cells with regard to features they have in common with other types of stem cells, such as embryonic, hematopoietic, or mesenchymal stem cells. In several studies, though they differed in methodology and technology, common features of stem cells have been specified, including neural stem cells [131-134]: First, stem cells proliferate in the presence of suitable growth factors. With regard to neural stem cells, EGF and FGF-2 have been identified as growth factors. Second, stem cells express genes of developmental signaling pathways. Of these, Shh, Notch, TGF-beta, Wnt, or JAK/STAT have been identified in neural stem cells. Third, stem cells interact with specific molecules of the extracellular matrix. Of these, integrins and cadherins have been identified in neural stem cells. Fourth, all types of stem cells express genes regulating transcription and translation, including genes for the regulation of the cell cycle, indicating their highly active state. Fifth, stem cells seem to have developed specialized mechanisms which protect them from "cell stress". Genes involved include transcripts for detoxification, DNA repair, protein folding and degradation.

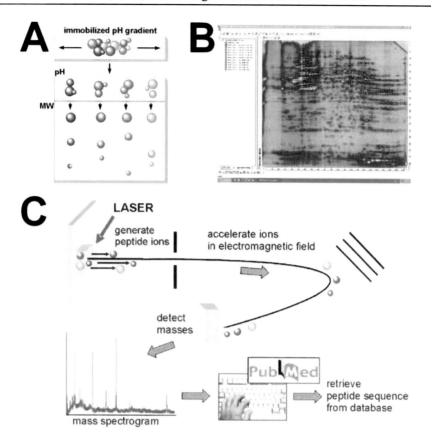

Fig. 5. Principle of the proteomic technique. (A) Schematic workflow of two-dimensional gel electrophoresis: In the first dimension, proteins are separated in immobilized pH gradient gels according to their isoelectric point. In the second dimension, proteins are separated on polyacrylamide gels according to their molecular weight. (B) Image analysis: Protein gels are stained and analyzed by a special software (here: Phoretix 2D Expression, Nonlinear Dynamics, Newcastle-upon-Tyne, UK) to detect spots, to quantify protein expression and to create image overlays. (C) Spot identification by mass spectrometry: Spots of interest are excised and digested. The resulting peptides are subjected to matrix-assisted laser desorption/ionization-time-of-flight (MALDI-TOF) mass spectrometry, where peptide ions are generated by a laser beam. Then the ions are accelerated in an electric field and the time is measured until they reach the mass detector. The resulting mass spectrogram combining mass and charge of the molecules is characteristic for a specific protein, the sequence of which can be retrieved from a database (modified from [142]).

The search for "stemness" genes, i. e. genes common to all stem cells, concentrated on the common functional properties of stem cells, which are multipotency and self-renewal [13, 7]. Concerning neural stem cells, it is of interest, which sets of genes are unique to these stem cells. Indeed, some unique genes appear to exist in neural stem cells which can be grouped functionally into the categories of transcriptional regulation, reaction to cellular growth, cell cycle regulation, oxidative metabolism, and signaling cascades [135, 136].

Proteomic Screening

Whereas the genomic and transcriptomic level are mainly responsible for storing the potential for all components of cell morphology and function, the actual "executive tasks" take place at the protein level. In analogy to the large-scale analysis of the genome and transcriptome, proteomics as the study of the proteome aim at describing and characterizing all proteins in a given sample [137-142].

Major technologies developed for proteomics include two-dimensional gel electrophoresis based on the separation of proteins according to their isoelectric point and molecular mass [143-145, 142] (Fig. 5), direct mass spectrometric approaches [146, 138, 117, 147, 139], and chip-based concepts of protein analysis [148-152]. In a broader sense, also high-throughput analysis of multiple surface antigens by fluorescence-activated cell sorting (FACS) may be subsumed by proteomic screening.

Although protein expression profiling has gained an emancipated position at the side of gene expression profiling, this subject is not free of obstacles and pitfalls. Technological shortcomings involve the poor resolution of hydrophobic proteins in two-dimensional gels, the cumbersome approach of mass spectrometry prohibiting its wide use, and when using a protein chip, the limited number of target sequences. Besides these technical limitations, also biological issues complicate the use of proteomics. For example, the dynamic range of protein expression is about 10^7, whereas the dynamic range of protein analytical methods seldom exceeds the range of 10^4 [153]. This means that it is nearly impossible to resolve both low-abundant and high-abundant proteins in the same experimental setup.

Moreover, posttranslational modifications of proteins influence the results of a specific proteomic experiment. For maintaining cell function, a large number of proteins is continuously modified by all sorts of biochemical reactions including phosphorylation, glycosylation, the addition of carbohydrate sidechains (methylation and acetylation), proteolytic cleavage, and sulfation [154]. Post-translational modifications are highly dynamic processes on the basis of dynamic equilibria, thus a proteomic profile only depicts a certain point of time in the history of development and differentiation of a cell. Keeping these limitations in mind, proteomics are an extremely useful tool. They enable the screening of hundreds or even thousands of target sequences at once, which principally allows to monitor changes in cellular molecular morphology and function.

Neural stem cells have been subjected to proteomic analysis with the aim to delineate characteristic proteins or protein expression patterns. Proteome inventories of neural stem cells [155, 156] laid the basis for functional analysis of highly complex processes such as differentiation [157-159] and cellular maturation [160] of neural stem cells. Due to the limited number of studies performed in this field, and due to technical differences between the various approaches, a successful identification of exclusive marker proteins has not been achieved in neural stem cells on the proteomic level. It appears more likely to attribute comprehensive protein patterns consisting of several hundred items to specific types of stem cells rather than to characterize them on the basis of individual proteins.

Supporting this concept, two recent studies have focused on surface membrane proteins of neurospheres [161, 162]. The authors constructed protein microarrays consisting of antibodies immobilized on activated glass or membrane surfaces. Using such microarrays, they found that characteristic patterns of membrane proteins exist in neurospheres, although none of the proteins identified on the neurosphere cell surface is uniquely expressed in neural stem cells. For example, CD15 (Lewis-X) is found on the surface of most neurospheres, but also on neutrophils, eosinophils, and some types of monocytes. Or, for example, CD133 is a protein which is more restricted to stem cells. However, it is not exclusively present in neural, but also exists in hematopoietic stem cells.

Compared to protein chips, a higher number of cell surface proteins can be investigated by fluorescence-activated cell sorting (FACS) analysis [163]. In principle, FACS analysis starts by incubating the cells of interest with antibodies specific to the surface antigen of interest. The antibodies are labeled with a fluorophore. When single labeled cells pass through a small capillary, each fluorescent signal can be counted. Coupling the device to a laser sorting system allows to collect the fraction of labeled cells. The combination of multiple surface markers can result in complex multiplexed systems consisting of cells stained by up to 10 or more markers which allow the isolation of neural stem cells from a heterogeneous mixture of cells [164, 73]. Of note, there is no single marker for neural stem cells available using this system, but the combination of a set of markers may give better results (Fig. 3). Moreover, for the definition of neural precursor cells it may be helpful that the surface markers appear to correlate well with the expression of certain subtypes of ion channels, such as Na^+, K^+, and Ca^{++} channels, and their respective electrophysiological properties, as revealed by the characteristic voltage-current diagrams [165, 45, 166, 73].

Conclusion

It is not possible to define a suitable marker specific for neural stem cells. However, several marker proteins are expressed in neural stem cells, indicating that neural stem cells do not represent a homogeneous population in the brain. Regional differences with regard to the gene and protein expression pattern of neural stem cells as well as their proliferation and differentiation behavior have been described [167, 168]. These properties of neural stem cells are compatible with the concept that several subtypes of neural stem cells exist in the brain which do not have the identical potential for proliferation and differentiation [169, 136]. Moreover, differences exist between the *in vitro* and *in vivo* situation. For example, the trilineage potential of neural stem cells which allows them to differentiate into neurons, astrocytes, and oligodendrocytes *in vitro* has not yet been confirmed *in vivo* [59]. On the other hand, it is well agreed that neural stem cells express markers within a developmental program which may define their status in time and space [15, 170, 56]. Thus, molecular signatures of neural stem cells appear to be specific only for a single anatomical location and a single point of time in development with regard to their actual functional status.

This heterogeneity in stem cell populations in the brain as reflected by different gene and protein expression patterns as well as divergent cell biological behavior may lead to a new definition of neural stem cells. This definition would go beyond functional aspects [15, 171] and integrate the systems biology aspect of respective expression patterns. This means that individual gene and protein expression patterns obtained by genomic, transcriptomic, or proteomic experiments should be used for the definition of specific subtypes of neural stem cells (Fig. 6). In this concept, the definition of neural stem cells is not based on the expression of an individual gene or protein, but rather on the pattern of the whole set of hundreds, or thousands, of genes and proteins. Future developments especially in the field of bioinformatics will allow an easier accession and comparison of large-scale datasets [172, 173, 115]. Thus this systems biology-based definition of stem cells and of their subtypes will become more practical and applicable in the every day use.

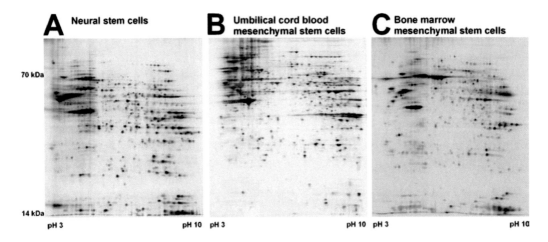

Fig. 6. Comparison of two-dimensional gel images of different types of stem cells. The data show a specific protein expression pattern for each of the stem cell types which is clearly distinct from the expression pattern of the others. (A) neural stem cells, data from [159], (B) mesenchymal stem cells from umbilical cord blood, data from [175], (C) mesenchymal stem cells from bone marrow, data from [176].

Acknowledgements

This work was supported by the German Ministry of Education and Research (BMBF) within the National Genome Research Network NGFN-2 (N3NV-S19T05) and the German Research Foundation (DFG, MA 2492/2-2).

References

[1]   Schleiden, M. J.; Schwann, T. (1838). Beiträge zur Phytogenesis. In: Müller, J. (Ed.). Archiv für Anatomie, *Physiologie und wissenschaftliche Medicin.* Berlin, Germany: Veit.

[2]   Virchow, R. (1858). *Die Cellularpathologie.* Berlin, Germany: August Hirschwald.

[3]   Golgi, C. (1903 (vol. I-III), 1929 (vol. IV post.)). *Opera Omnia.* Milano, Italy: Hoepli Editore.

[4]   Ramón y Cajal, S. (1909 (vol. I), 1911 (vol. II)). H*istologie du Système Nerveux de l'Homme et des Vertébrés.* Paris: Maloine.

[5]   Sauer, F. C. (1935). Mitosis in the neural tube. *J Comp Neurol,* 62, 377-405.

[6]   Gerhart, J. (1999). 1998 Warkany lecture: signaling pathways in development. *Teratology,* 60, 226-239.

[7] Imitola, J.; Snyder, E. Y.; Khoury, S. J. (2003). Genetic programs and responses of neural stem/progenitor cells during demyelination: potential insights into repair mechanisms in multiple sclerosis. *Physiol Genomics*, 14, 171-197.

[8] Imitola, J.; Park, K. I.; Teng, Y. D.; Nisim, S.; Lachyankar, M.; Ourednik, J.; Mueller, F. J.; Yiou, R.; Atala, A.; Sidman, R. L.; Tuszynski, M.; Khoury, S. J.; Snyder, E. Y. (2004). Stem cells: cross-talk and developmental programs. *Philos Trans R Soc Lond B Biol Sci*, 359, 823-837.

[9] Hall, P. A.; Watt, F. M. (1989). Stem cells: the generation and maintenance of cellular diversity. *Development*, 106, 619-633.

[10] Potten, C. S.; Loeffler, M. (1990). Stem cells: attributes, cycles, spirals, pitfalls and uncertainties. Lessons for and from the crypt. *Development*, 110, 1001-1020.

[11] Weissman, I. L. (2000). Stem cells: units of development, units of regeneration, and units in evolution. *Cell*, 100, 157-168.

[12] Temple, S.; Qian, X. (1996). Vertebrate neural progenitor cells: subtypes and regulation. *Curr Opin Neurobiol*, 6, 11-17.

[13] Gage, F. H. (2000). Mammalian neural stem cells. *Science*, 287, 1433-1438.

[14] Gage, F. H. (2002). Neurogenesis in the adult brain. *J Neurosci*, 22, 612-613.

[15] Rakic, P. (2002). Adult neurogenesis in mammals: an identity crisis. *J Neurosci,* 22, 614-618.

[16] Galli, R.; Gritti, A.; Bonfanti, L.; Vescovi, A. L. (2003). Neural stem cells: an overview. *Circ Res*, 92, 598-608.

[17] Altman, J.; Das, G. D. (1965). Autoradiographic and histological evidence of postnatal hippocampal neurogenesis in rats. *J Comp Neurol*, 124, 319-335.

[18] Gage, F. H.; Coates, P. W.; Palmer, T. D.; Kuhn, H. G.; Fisher, L. J.; Suhonen, J. O.; Peterson, D. A.; Suhr, S. T.; Ray, J. (1995). Survival and differentiation of adult neuronal progenitor cells transplanted to the adult brain. *Proc Natl Acad Sci USA*, 92, 11879-11883.

[19] Eriksson, P. S.; Perfilieva, E.; Bjork-Eriksson, T.; Alborn, A. M.; Nordborg, C.; Peterson, D. A.; Gage, F. H. (1998). Neurogenesis in the adult human hippocampus. *Nat Med*, 4, 1313-1317.

[20] Magavi, S. S.; Leavitt, B. R.; Macklis, J. D. (2000). Induction of neurogenesis in the neocortex of adult mice. *Nature*, 405, 951-955.

[21] Roy, N. S.; Wang, S.; Jiang, L.; Kang, J.; Benraiss, A.; Harrison-Restelli, C.; Fraser, R. A.; Couldwell, W. T.; Kawaguchi, A.; Okano, H.; Nedergaard, M.; Goldman, S. A. (2000). In vitro neurogenesis by progenitor cells isolated from the adult human hippocampus. *Nat Med*, 6, 271-277.

[22] Morshead, C. M.; Reynolds, B. A.; Craig, C. G.; McBurney, M. W.; Staines, W. A.; Morassutti, D.; Weiss, S.; van der Kooy, D. (1994). Neural stem cells in the adult mammalian forebrain: a relatively quiescent subpopulation of subependymal cells. *Neuron*, 13, 1071-1082.

[23] Levison, S. W.; Goldman, J. E. (1997). Multipotential and lineage restricted precursors coexist in the mammalian perinatal subventricular zone. *J Neurosci Res*, 48, 83-94.

[24] Doetsch, F.; Caille, I.; Lim, D. A.; Garcia-Verdugo, J. M.; Alvarez-Buylla, A. (1999). Subventricular zone astrocytes are neural stem cells in the adult mammalian brain. *Cell*, 97, 703-716.

[25] Ben-Hur, T.; Rogister, B.; Murray, K.; Rougon, G.; Dubois-Dalcq, M. (1998). Growth and fate of PSA-NCAM+ precursors of the postnatal brain. *J Neurosci*, 18, 5777-5788.

[26] Marmur, R.; Mabie, P. C.; Gokhan, S.; Song, Q.; Kessler, J. A.; Mehler, M. F. (1998). Isolation and developmental characterization of cerebral cortical multipotent progenitors. *Dev Biol*, 204, 577-591.

[27] Arsenijevic, Y.; Villemure, J. G.; Brunet, J. F.; Bloch, J. J.; Deglon, N.; Kostic, C.; Zurn, A.; Aebischer, P. (2001). Isolation of multipotent neural precursors residing in the cortex of the adult human brain. *Exp Neurol*, 170, 48-62.

[28] Cai, J.; Wu, Y.; Mirua, T.; Pierce, J. L.; Lucero, M. T.; Albertine, K. H.; Spangrude, G. J.; Rao, M. S. (2002). Properties of a fetal multipotent neural stem cell (NEP cell). *Dev Biol*, 251, 221-240.

[29] Zhao, M.; Momma, S.; Delfani, K.; Carlen, M.; Cassidy, R. M.; Johansson, C. B.; Brismar, H.; Shupliakov, O.; Frisen, J.; Janson, A. M. (2003). Evidence for neurogenesis in the adult mammalian substantia nigra. *Proc Natl Acad Sci* USA, 100, 7925-7930.

[30] Kukekov, V. G.; Laywell, E. D.; Suslov, O.; Davies, K.; Scheffler, B.; Thomas, L. B.; O'Brien, T. F.; Kusakabe, M.; Steindler, D. A. (1999). Multipotent stem/ progenitor cells with similar properties arise from two neurogenic regions of adult human brain. *Exp Neurol*, 156, 333-344.

[31] Johansson, C. B.; Momma, S.; Clarke, D. L.; Risling, M.; Lendahl, U.; Frisen, J. (1999). Identification of a neural stem cell in the adult mammalian central nervous system. *Cell*, 96, 25-34.

[32] Johansson, C. B.; Svensson, M.; Wallstedt, L.; Janson, A. M.; Frisen, J. (1999). Neural stem cells in the adult human brain. *Exp Cell Res*, 253, 733-736.

[33] Laywell, E. D.; Rakic, P.; Kukekov, V. G.; Holland, E. C.; Steindler, D. A. (2000). Identification of a multipotent astrocytic stem cell in the immature and adult mouse brain. *Proc Natl Acad Sci* U S A, 97, 13883-13888.

[34] Doetsch, F. (2003). The glial identity of neural stem cells. *Nat Neurosci*, 6, 1127-1134.

[35] Malatesta, P.; Hartfuss, E.; Götz, M. (2000). Isolation of radial glial cells by fluorescent-activated cell sorting reveals a neuronal lineage. *Development*, 127, 5253-5263.

[36] Miyata, T.; Kawaguchi, A.; Okano, H.; Ogawa, M. (2001). Asymmetric inheritance of radial glial fibers by cortical neurons. *Neuron*, 31, 727-741.

[37] Noctor, S. C.; Flint, A. C.; Weissman, T. A.; Wong, W. S.; Clinton, B. K.; Kriegstein, A. R. (2002). Dividing precursor cells of the embryonic cortical ventricular zone have morphological and molecular characteristics of radial glia. J *Neurosci*, 22, 3161-3173.

[38] Malatesta, P.; Hack, M. A.; Hartfuss, E.; Kettenmann, H.; Klinkert, W.; Kirchhoff, F.; Götz, M. (2003). Neuronal or glial progeny: regional differences in radial glia fate. *Neuron*, 37, 751-764.

[39] Goldman, S. A. (1998). Adult neurogenesis: from canaries to the clinic. *J Neurobiol*, 36, 267-286.

[40] Okano, H. (2002). Neural stem cells: progression of basic research and perspective for clinical application. *Keio J Med*, 51, 115-128.

[41] Björklund, A.; Lindvall, O. (2000). Cell replacement therapies for central nervous system disorders. *Nat Neurosci*, 3, 537-544.

[42] Kokaia, Z.; Lindvall, O. (2003). Neurogenesis after ischaemic brain insults. *Curr Opin Neurobiol*, 13, 127-132.

[43] Ostenfeld, T.; Svendsen, C. N. (2003). Recent advances in stem cell neurobiology. *Adv Tech Stand Neurosurg*, 28, 3-89.

[44] Lie, D. C.; Song, H.; Colamarino, S. A.; Ming, G. L.; Gage, F. H. (2004). Neurogenesis in the adult brain: new strategies for central nervous system diseases. *Annu Rev Pharmacol Toxicol*, 44, 399-421.

[45] van Praag, H.; Schinder, A. F.; Christie, B. R.; Toni, N.; Palmer, T. D.; Gage, F. H. (2002). Functional neurogenesis in the adult hippocampus. *Nature*, 415, 1030-1034.

[46] Wernig, M.; Benninger, F.; Schmandt, T.; Rade, M.; Tucker, K. L.; Bussow, H.; Beck, H.; Brüstle, O. (2004). Functional integration of embryonic stem cell-derived neurons in vivo. *J Neurosci*, 24, 5258-5268.

[47] Mezey, E.; Chandross, K. J.; Harta, G.; Maki, R. A.; McKercher, S. R. (2000). Turning blood into brain: cells bearing neuronal antigens generated in vivo from bone marrow. *Science*, 290, 1779-1782.

[48] Priller, J.; Persons, D. A.; Klett, F. F.; Kempermann, G.; Kreutzberg, G. W.; Dirnagl, U. (2001). Neogenesis of cerebellar Purkinje neurons from gene-marked bone marrow cells in vivo. *J Cell Biol*, 155, 733-738.

[49] Sanchez-Ramos, J. R. (2002). Neural cells derived from adult bone marrow and umbilical cord blood. *J Neurosci Res*, 69, 880-893.

[50] Jin, K.; Mao, X. O.; Batteur, S.; Sun, Y.; Greenberg, D. A. (2003). Induction of neuronal markers in bone marrow cells: differential effects of growth factors and patterns of intracellular expression. *Exp Neurol*, 184, 78-89.

[51] Wislet-Gendebien, S.; Hans, G.; Leprince, P.; Rigo, J. M.; Moonen, G.; Rogister, B. (2005). Plasticity of cultured mesenchymal stem cells: switch from nestin-positive to excitable neuron-like phenotype. *Stem Cells*, 23, 392-402.

[52] McGuckin, C. P.; Forraz, N.; Allouard, Q.; Pettengell, R. (2004). Umbilical cord blood stem cells can expand hematopoietic and neuroglial progenitors in vitro. *Exp Cell Res*, 295, 350-359.

[53] U.S. Department of Health and Human Services (2001). Stem Cells: Scientific Progress and Future Research Directions [online]. Available from: *http://stemcells.nih.gov/info/scireport/*.

[54] Kornblum, H. I.; Geschwind, D. H. (2001). Molecular markers in CNS stem cell research: hitting a moving target. *Nat Rev Neurosci*, 2, 843-846.

[55] Goldman, J. E. (2003). What are the characteristics of cycling cells in the adult central nervous system? *J Cell Biochem*, 88, 20-23.

[56] Rao, M. (2004). Stem and precursor cells in the nervous system. *J Neurotrauma*, 21, 415-427.

[57] Rao, M. S. (2004). Stem sense: A proposal for the classification of stem cells. *Stem Cells Dev*, 13, 452-455.

[58] Gabay, L.; Lowell, S.; Rubin, L. L.; Anderson, D. J. (2003). Deregulation of dorsoventral patterning by FGF confers trilineage differentiation capacity on CNS stem cells in vitro. *Neuron*, 40, 485-499.

[59] Stiles, C. D. (2003). Lost in space: misregulated positional cues create tripotent neural progenitors in cell culture. *Neuron*, 40, 447-449.

[60] Reynolds, B. A.; Tetzlaff, W.; Weiss, S. (1992). A multipotent EGF-responsive striatal embryonic progenitor cell produces neurons and astrocytes. *J Neurosci*, 12, 4565-4574.

[61] Reynolds, B. A.; Weiss, S. (1992). Generation of neurons and astrocytes from isolated cells of the adult mammalian central nervous system. *Science*, 255, 1707-1710.

[62] Ray, J.; Peterson, D. A.; Schinstine, M.; Gage, F. H. (1993). Proliferation, differentiation, and long-term culture of primary hippocampal neurons. *Proc Natl Acad Sci* USA, 90, 3602-3606.

[63] Reynolds, B. A.; Rietze, R. (2005). Neural stem cells and neurospheres -- re-evaluating the relationship. *Nat Meth*, 2, 333-336.

[64] Weissman, I. L.; Anderson, D. J.; Gage, F. (2001). Stem and progenitor cells: origins, phenotypes, lineage commitments, and transdifferentiations. *Annu Rev Cell Dev Biol*, 17, 387-403.

[65] Bonnet, D. (2002). Haematopoietic stem cells. *J Pathol*, 197, 430-440.

[66] Jackson, K. A.; Majka, S. M.; Wulf, G. G.; Goodell, M. A. (2002). Stem cells: a minireview. *J Cell Biochem Suppl*, 38, 1-6.

[67] Eiges, R.; Benvenisty, N. (2002). A molecular view on pluripotent stem cells. *FEBS Lett*, 529, 135-141.

[68] Bazan, E.; Alonso, F. J.; Redondo, C.; Lopez-Toledano, M. A.; Alfaro, J. M.; Reimers, D.; Herranz, A. S.; Paino, C. L.; Serrano, A. B.; Cobacho, N.; Caso, E.; Lobo, M. V. (2004). In vitro and in vivo characterization of neural stem cells. *Histol Histopathol*, 19, 1261-1275.

[69] Lendahl, U.; Zimmerman, L. B.; McKay, R. D. (1990). CNS stem cells express a new class of intermediate filament protein. *Cell*, 60, 585-595.

[70] Lendahl, U. (1997). Gene regulation in the formation of the central nervous system. *Acta Paediatr Suppl*, 422, 8-11.

[71] Wiese, C.; Rolletschek, A.; Kania, G.; Blyszczuk, P.; Tarasov, K. V.; Tarasova, Y.; Wersto, R. P.; Boheler, K. R.; Wobus, A. M. (2004). Nestin expression--a property of multi-lineage progenitor cells? *Cell Mol Life Sci*, 61, 2510-2522.

[72] Fukuda, S.; Kato, F.; Tozuka, Y.; Yamaguchi, M.; Miyamoto, Y.; Hisatsune, T. (2003). Two distinct subpopulations of nestin-positive cells in adult mouse dentate gyrus. *J Neurosci*, 23, 9357-9366.

[73] Maric, D.; Barker, J. L. (2004). Neural stem cells redefined: a FACS perspective. *Mol Neurobiol*, 30, 49-76.

[74] Dolbeare, F. (1995). Bromodeoxyuridine: a diagnostic tool in biology and medicine, Part I: Historical perspectives, histochemical methods and cell kinetics. *Histochem J*, 27, 339-369.

[75] Nowakowski, R. S.; Lewin, S. B.; Miller, M. W. (1989). Bromodeoxyuridine immunohistochemical determination of the lengths of the cell cycle and the DNA-synthetic phase for an anatomically defined population. *J Neurocytol*, 18, 311-318.

[76] Doetsch, F.; Garcia-Verdugo, J. M.; Alvarez-Buylla, A. (1999). Regeneration of a germinal layer in the adult mammalian brain. *Proc Natl Acad Sci* USA, 96, 11619-11624.

[77] Cooper-Kuhn, C. M.; Kuhn, H. G. (2002). Is it all DNA repair? Methodological considerations for detecting neurogenesis in the adult brain. *Brain Res Dev Brain Res*, 134, 13-21.

[78] Maslov, A. Y.; Barone, T. A.; Plunkett, R. J.; Pruitt, S. C. (2004). Neural stem cell detection, characterization, and age-related changes in the subventricular zone of mice. *J Neurosci*, 24, 1726-1733.

[79] Barres, B. A. (1999). A new role for glia: generation of neurons! Cell, 97, 667-670.

[80] Kimelberg, H. K. (2004). The problem of astrocyte identity. *Neurochem Int*, 45, 191-202.

[81] Rakic, P. (1972). Mode of cell migration to the superficial layers of fetal monkey neocortex. *J Comp Neurol*, 145, 61-83.

[82] Levitt, P.; Rakic, P. (1980). Immunoperoxidase localization of glial fibrillary acidic protein in radial glial cells and astrocytes of the developing rhesus monkey brain. *J Comp Neurol*, 193, 815-840.

[83] Gregg, C. T.; Chojnacki, A. K.; Weiss, S. (2002). Radial glial cells as neuronal precursors: the next generation? *J Neurosci Res*, 69, 708-713.

[84] Gregg, C.; Weiss, S. (2003). Generation of functional radial glial cells by embryonic and adult forebrain neural stem cells. *J Neurosci*, 23, 11587-11601.

[85] Doetsch, F.; Garcia-Verdugo, J. M.; Alvarez-Buylla, A. (1997). Cellular composition and three-dimensional organization of the subventricular germinal zone in the adult mammalian brain. *J Neurosci*, 17, 5046-5061.

[86] Momma, S.; Johansson, C. B.; Frisen, J. (2000). Get to know your stem cells. *Curr Opin Neurobiol*, 10, 45-49.

[87] Alvarez-Buylla, A.; Lim, D. A. (2004). For the long run: maintaining germinal niches in the adult brain. *Neuron*, 41, 683-686.

[88] Rakic, P. (1982). Early developmental events: cell lineages, acquisition of neuronal positions, and areal and laminar development. *Neurosci Res Program Bull*, 20, 439-451.

[89] Heins, N.; Malatesta, P.; Cecconi, F.; Nakafuku, M.; Tucker, K. L.; Hack, M. A.; Chapouton, P.; Barde, Y. A.; Götz, M. (2002). Glial cells generate neurons: the role of the transcription factor Pax6. *Nat Neurosci*, 5, 308-315.

[90] Hack, M. A.; Saghatelyan, A.; de Chevigny, A.; Pfeifer, A.; Ashery-Padan, R.; Lledo, P. M.; Gotz, M. (2005). Neuronal fate determinants of adult olfactory bulb neurogenesis. *Nat Neurosci.*

[91] Arendt, D. (2003). Evolution of eyes and photoreceptor cell types. *Int J Dev Biol*, 47, 563-571.

[92] Schonhoff, S. E.; Giel-Moloney, M.; Leiter, A. B. (2004). Minireview: Development and differentiation of gut endocrine cells. *Endocrinology*, 145, 2639-2644.

[93] Kaneko, Y.; Sakakibara, S.; Imai, T.; Suzuki, A.; Nakamura, Y.; Sawamoto, K.; Ogawa, Y.; Toyama, Y.; Miyata, T.; Okano, H. (2000). Musashi1: an evolutionally conserved marker for CNS progenitor cells including neural stem cells. *Dev Neurosci*, 22, 139-153.

[94] Keyoung, H. M.; Roy, N. S.; Benraiss, A.; Louissaint, A., Jr.; Suzuki, A.; Hashimoto, M.; Rashbaum, W. K.; Okano, H.; Goldman, S. A. (2001). High-yield selection and extraction of two promoter-defined phenotypes of neural stem cells from the fetal human brain. *Nat Biotechnol*, 19, 843-850.

[95] Sakakibara, S.; Nakamura, Y.; Yoshida, T.; Shibata, S.; Koike, M.; Takano, H.; Ueda, S.; Uchiyama, Y.; Noda, T.; Okano, H. (2002). RNA-binding protein Musashi family: roles for CNS stem cells and a subpopulation of ependymal cells revealed by targeted disruption and antisense ablation. *Proc Natl Acad Sci* USA, 99, 15194-15199.

[96] Kayahara, T.; Sawada, M.; Takaishi, S.; Fukui, H.; Seno, H.; Fukuzawa, H.; Suzuki, K.; Hiai, H.; Kageyama, R.; Okano, H.; Chiba, T. (2003). Candidate markers for stem and early progenitor cells, Musashi-1 and Hes1, are expressed in crypt base columnar cells of mouse small intestine. *FEBS Lett*, 535, 131-135.

[97] Francis, F.; Koulakoff, A.; Boucher, D.; Chafey, P.; Schaar, B.; Vinet, M. C.; Friocourt, G.; McDonnell, N.; Reiner, O.; Kahn, A.; McConnell, S. K.; Berwald-Netter, Y.; Denoulet, P.; Chelly, J. (1999). Doublecortin is a developmentally regulated, microtubule-associated protein expressed in migrating and differentiating neurons. *Neuron*, 23, 247-256.

[98] Brown, J. P.; Couillard-Despres, S.; Cooper-Kuhn, C. M.; Winkler, J.; Aigner, L.; Kuhn, H. G. (2003). Transient expression of doublecortin during adult neurogenesis. *J Comp Neurol*, 467, 1-10.

[99] Couillard-Despres, S.; Winner, B.; Schaubeck, S.; Aigner, R.; Vroemen, M.; Weidner, N.; Bogdahn, U.; Winkler, J.; Kuhn, H. G.; Aigner, L. (2005). Doublecortin expression levels in adult brain reflect neurogenesis. *Eur J Neurosci*, 21, 1-14.

[100] Pevny, L.; Placzek, M. (2005). SOX genes and neural progenitor identity. *Curr Opin Neurobiol*, 15, 7-13.

[101] Fargeas, C. A.; Corbeil, D.; Huttner, W. B. (2003). AC133 antigen, CD133, prominin-1, prominin-2, etc.: prominin family gene products in need of a rational nomenclature. *Stem Cells*, 21, 506-508.

[102] Scheel, J.; Von Brevern, M. C.; Horlein, A.; Fischer, A.; Schneider, A.; Bach, A. (2002). Yellow pages to the transcriptome. *Pharmacogenomics*, 3, 791-807.

[103] Brazma, A.; Hingamp, P.; Quackenbush, J.; Sherlock, G.; Spellman, P.; Stoeckert, C.; Aach, J.; Ansorge, W.; Ball, C. A.; Causton, H. C.; Gaasterland, T.; Glenisson, P.; Holstege, F. C.; Kim, I. F.; Markowitz, V.; Matese, J. C.; Parkinson, H.; Robinson, A.; Sarkans, U.; Schulze-Kremer, S.; Stewart, J.; Taylor, R.; Vilo, J.; Vingron, M. (2001). Minimum information about a microarray experiment (MIAME)-toward standards for microarray data. *Nat Genet*, 29, 365-371.

[104] Schena, M. (1996). Genome analysis with gene expression microarrays. Bioessays, 18, 427-431.

[105] Lee, P. S.; Lee, K. H. (2000). Genomic analysis. *Curr Opin Biotechnol*, 11, 171-175.

[106] Fadiel, A.; Naftolin, F. (2003). Microarray applications and challenges: a vast array of possibilities. *Int Arch Biosci*, 1111-1121.

[107] Choudhuri, S. (2004). Microarrays in biology and medicine. J Biochem Mol Toxicol, 18, 171-179.

[108] Duggan, D. J.; Bittner, M.; Chen, Y.; Meltzer, P.; Trent, J. M. (1999). Expression profiling using cDNA microarrays. *Nat Genet*, 21, 10-14.

[109] Schulze, A.; Downward, J. (2001). Navigating gene expression using microarrays-- a technology review. *Nat Cell Biol*, 3, E190-195.

[110] Dudoit, S.; Yang, Y. H.; Callow, M. J.; Speed, T. P. (2002). Statistical methods for identifying differentially expressed genes in replicated cDNA microarray experiments. *Statistica Sinica*, 12, 111-139.

[111] Yang, Y. H.; Speed, T. (2002). Design issues for cDNA microarray experiments. *Nat Rev Genet*, 3, 579-588.

[112] Smyth, G. K.; Yang, Y. H.; Speed, T. (2003). Statistical issues in cDNA microarray data analysis. *Methods Mol Biol*, 224, 111-136.

[113] Thieffry, D. (1999). From global expression data to gene networks. *Bioessays*, 21, 895-899.

[114] Wu, T. D. (2001). Analysing gene expression data from DNA microarrays to identify candidate genes. *J Pathol*, 195, 53-65.

[115] Kanehisa, M.; Bork, P. (2003). Bioinformatics in the post-sequence era. *Nat Genet*, 33 Suppl, 305-310.

[116] Maurer, M. H. (2004). The path to enlightenment: making sense of genomic and proteomic information. *Genomics Proteomics Bioinformatics*, 2, 123-131.

[117] Aebersold, R.; Mann, M. (2003). Mass spectrometry-based proteomics. *Nature*, 422, 198-207.

[118] Aggarwal, K.; Lee, K. H. (2003). Functional genomics and proteomics as a foundation for systems biology. *Briefings in Functional Genomics and Proteomics*, 2, 175-184.

[119] Patterson, S. D.; Aebersold, R. H. (2003). Proteomics: the first decade and beyond. *Nat Genet*, 33 Suppl, 311-323.

[120] Smith, L.; Greenfield, A. (2003). DNA microarrays and development. *Hum Mol Genet*, 12 Spec No 1, R1-8.

[121] Wen, X.; Fuhrman, S.; Michaels, G. S.; Carr, D. B.; Smith, S.; Barker, J. L.; Somogyi, R. (1998). Large-scale temporal gene expression mapping of central nervous system development. *Proc Natl Acad Sci* USA, 95, 334-339.

[122] Gurok, U.; Steinhoff, C.; Lipkowitz, B.; Ropers, H. H.; Scharff, C.; Nuber, U. A. (2004). Gene expression changes in the course of neural progenitor cell differentiation. *J Neurosci*, 24, 5982-6002.

[123] Loring, J. F.; Porter, J. G.; Seilhammer, J.; Kaser, M. R.; Wesselschmidt, R. (2001). A gene expression profile of embryonic stem cells and embryonic stem cell-derived neurons. *Restor Neurol Neurosci*, 18, 81-88.

[124] Zhou, F. C.; Duguid, J. R.; Edenberg, H. J.; McClintick, J.; Young, P.; Nelson, P. (2001). DNA microarray analysis of differential gene expression of 6-year-old rat neural striatal progenitor cells during early differentiation. *Restor Neurol Neurosci*, 18, 95-104.

[125] Wright, L. S.; Li, J.; Caldwell, M. A.; Wallace, K.; Johnson, J. A.; Svendsen, C. N. (2003). Gene expression in human neural stem cells: effects of leukemia inhibitory factor. *J Neurochem*, 86, 179-195.

[126] Huttner, W. B.; Brand, M. (1997). Asymmetric division and polarity of neuroepithelial cells. *Curr Opin Neurobiol*, 7, 29-39.

[127] Chenn, A.; Zhang, Y. A.; Chang, B. T.; McConnell, S. K. (1998). Intrinsic polarity of mammalian neuroepithelial cells. *Mol Cell Neurosci*, 11, 183-193.

[128] Jan, Y. N.; Jan, L. Y. (1998). Asymmetric cell division. *Nature*, 392, 775-778.

[129] Zhong, W. (2003). Diversifying neural cells through order of birth and asymmetry of division. Neuron, 37, 11-14.

[130] Ahn, J. I.; Lee, K. H.; Shin, D. M.; Shim, J. W.; Lee, J. S.; Chang, S. Y.; Lee, Y. S.; Brownstein, M. J.; Lee, S. H. (2004). Comprehensive transcriptome analysis of differentiation of embryonic stem cells into midbrain and hindbrain neurons. *Dev Biol*, 265, 491-501.

[131] Burns, C. E.; Zon, L. I. (2002). Portrait of a stem cell. *Dev Cell*, 3, 612-613.

[132] Ivanova, N. B.; Dimos, J. T.; Schaniel, C.; Hackney, J. A.; Moore, K. A.; Lemischka, I. R. (2002). A stem cell molecular signature. *Science*, 298, 601-604.

[133] Ramalho-Santos, M.; Yoon, S.; Matsuzaki, Y.; Mulligan, R. C.; Melton, D. A. (2002). "Stemness": transcriptional profiling of embryonic and adult stem cells. *Science*, 298, 597-600.

[134] Li, L.; Akashi, K. (2003). Unraveling the molecular components and genetic blueprints of stem cells. *Biotechniques*, 35, 1233-1239.

[135] Geschwind, D. H.; Ou, J.; Easterday, M. C.; Dougherty, J. D.; Jackson, R. L.; Chen, Z.; Antoine, H.; Terskikh, A.; Weissman, I. L.; Nelson, S. F.; Kornblum, H. I. (2001). A genetic analysis of neural progenitor differentiation. *Neuron*, 29, 325-339.

[136] D'Amour, K. A.; Gage, F. H. (2003). Genetic and functional differences between multipotent neural and pluripotent embryonic stem cells. *Proc Natl Acad Sci* USA, 100 Suppl 1, 11866-11872.

[137] Lee, K. H. (2001). Proteomics: a technology-driven and technology-limited discovery science. *Trends Biotechnol*, 19, 217-222.

[138] Mann, M.; Hendrickson, R. C.; Pandey, A. (2001). Analysis of proteins and proteomes by mass spectrometry. *Annu Rev Biochem*, 70, 437-473.

[139] Freeman, W. M.; Hemby, S. E. (2004). Proteomics for protein expression profiling in neuroscience. *Neurochem Res*, 29, 1065-1081.

[140] Kim, S. I.; Voshol, H.; van Oostrum, J.; Hastings, T. G.; Cascio, M.; Glucksman, M. J. (2004). Neuroproteomics: expression profiling of the brain's proteomes in health and disease. *Neurochem Res*, 29, 1317-1331.

[141] Righetti, P. G.; Campostrini, N.; Pascali, J.; Hamdan, M.; Astner, H. (2004). Quantitative proteomics: a review of different methodologies. *Eur J Mass Spectrom* (Chichester, Eng), 10, 335-348.

[142] Maurer, M. H.; Kuschinsky, W. (2008). Proteomics. In: Lajtha, A. (Ed.). *Handbook of Neurochemistry and Molecular Neurobiology*. (3rd ed., in press). New York: Springer.

[143] Ong, S. E.; Pandey, A. (2001). An evaluation of the use of two-dimensional gel electrophoresis in proteomics. *Biomol Eng*, 18, 195-205.

[144] Rabilloud, T. (2002). Two-dimensional gel electrophoresis in proteomics: old, old fashioned, but it still climbs up the mountains. *Proteomics*, 2, 3-10.

[145] Görg, A.; Weiss, W.; Dunn, M. J. (2004). Current two-dimensional electrophoresis technology for proteomics. Proteomics, 4, 3665-3685.

[146] Bakhtiar, R.; Nelson, R. W. (2001). Mass spectrometry of the proteome. *Mol Pharmacol*, 60, 405-415.

[147] Davidsson, P.; Brinkmalm, A.; Karlsson, G.; Persson, R.; Lindbjer, M.; Puchades, M.; Folkesson, S.; Paulson, L.; Dahl, A.; Rymo, L.; Silberring, J.; Ekman, R.; Blennow, K. (2003). Clinical mass spectrometry in neuroscience. Proteomics and peptidomics. *Cell Mol Biol* (Noisy-le-grand), 49, 681-688.

[148] Nelson, R. W.; Nedelkov, D.; Tubbs, K. A. (2000). Biosensor chip mass spectrometry: a chip-based proteomics approach. *Electrophoresis*, 21, 1155-1163.

[149] Jenkins, R. E.; Pennington, S. R. (2001). Arrays for protein expression profiling: towards a viable alternative to two-dimensional gel electrophoresis? *Proteomics*, 1, 13-29.

[150] Fung, E. T.; Enderwick, C. (2002). ProteinChip clinical proteomics: computational challenges and solutions. *Biotechniques*, Suppl, 34-38, 40-31.

[151] James, P. (2002). Chips for proteomics: a new tool or just hype? *Biotechniques*, Suppl, 4-10, 12-13.

[152] Vonderwülbecke, S.; Cleverley, S.; Weinberger, S. R.; Wiesner, A. (2005). Protein quantification by the SELDI-TOF-MS-based ProteinChip(R) System. *Nat Meth*, 2, 393-395.

[153] Kusnezow, W.; Hoheisel, J. D. (2002). Antibody microarrays: promises and problems. *Biotechniques*, Suppl, 14-23.

[154] Mann, M.; Jensen, O. N. (2003). Proteomic analysis of post-translational modifications. *Nat Biotechnol*, 21, 255-261.

[155] Maurer, M. H.; Feldmann, R. E., Jr.; Fütterer, C. D.; Kuschinsky, W. (2003). The proteome of neural stem cells from adult rat hippocampus. *Proteome Sci*, 1, 4.

[156] Unwin, R. D.; Gaskell, S. J.; Evans, C. A.; Whetton, A. D. (2003). The potential for proteomic definition of stem cell populations. *Exp Hematol*, 31, 1147-1159.

[157] Pearce, A.; Svendsen, C. N. (1999). Characterisation of stem cell expression using two-dimensional electrophoresis. *Electrophoresis*, 20, 969-970.

[158] Guo, X.; Ying, W.; Wan, J.; Hu, Z.; Qian, X.; Zhang, H.; He, F. (2001). Proteomic characterization of early-stage differentiation of mouse embryonic stem cells into neural cells induced by all-trans retinoic acid in vitro. *Electrophoresis*, 22, 3067-3075.

[159] Maurer, M. H.; Feldmann, R. E.; Fütterer, C. D.; Butlin, J.; Kuschinsky, W. (2004). Comprehensive proteome expression profiling of undifferentiated vs. differentiated neural stem cells from adult rat hippocampus. *Neurochem Res*, 29, 1129-1144.

[160] Taoka, M.; Wakamiya, A.; Nakayama, H.; Isobe, T. (2000). Protein profiling of rat cerebella during development. *Electrophoresis*, 21, 1872-1879.

[161] Ko, I. K.; Kato, K.; Iwata, H. (2005). Parallel analysis of multiple surface markers expressed on rat neural stem cells using antibody microarrays. *Biomaterials*, 26, 4882-4891.

[162] Ko, I. K.; Kato, K.; Iwata, H. (2005). Antibody microarray for correlating cell phenotype with surface marker. *Biomaterials*, 26, 687-696.

[163] Silverstein, A. M. (2004). Labeled antigens and antibodies: the evolution of magic markers and magic bullets. *Nat Immunol*, 5, 1211-1217.

[164] Uchida, N.; Buck, D. W.; He, D.; Reitsma, M. J.; Masek, M.; Phan, T. V.; Tsukamoto, A. S.; Gage, F. H.; Weissman, I. L. (2000). Direct isolation of human central nervous system stem cells. *Proc Natl Acad Sci* USA, 97, 14720-14725.

[165] Piper, D. R.; Mujtaba, T.; Rao, M. S.; Lucero, M. T. (2000). Immunocytochemical and physiological characterization of a population of cultured human neural precursors. *J Neurophysiol*, 84, 534-548.

[166] Cai, J.; Cheng, A.; Luo, Y.; Lu, C.; Mattson, M. P.; Rao, M. S.; Furukawa, K. (2004). Membrane properties of rat embryonic multipotent neural stem cells. *J Neurochem*, 88, 212-226.

[167] Hitoshi, S.; Tropepe, V.; Ekker, M.; van der Kooy, D. (2002). Neural stem cell lineages are regionally specified, but not committed, within distinct compartments of the developing brain. *Development*, 129, 233-244.

[168] Ostenfeld, T.; Joly, E.; Tai, Y. T.; Peters, A.; Caldwell, M.; Jauniaux, E.; Svendsen, C. N. (2002). Regional specification of rodent and human neurospheres. *Brain Res Dev Brain Res*, 134, 43-55.

[169] D'Amour, K. A.; Gage, F. H. (2002). Are somatic stem cells pluripotent or lineage-restricted? *Nat Med*, 8, 213-214.

[170] Morshead, C. M.; van der Kooy, D. (2004). Disguising adult neural stem cells. *Curr Opin Neurobiol*, 14, 125-131.

[171] Doetsch, F.; Hen, R. (2005). Young and excitable: the function of new neurons in the adult mammalian brain. *Curr Opin Neurobiol*, 15, 121-128.

[172] Brown, P. O.; Botstein, D. (1999). Exploring the new world of the genome with DNA microarrays. *Nat Genet,* 21, 33-37.

[173] Achard, F.; Vaysseix, G.; Barillot, E. (2001). XML, bioinformatics and data integration. *Bioinformatics*, 17, 115-125.

[174] Moyer, M. P.; Johnson, R. A.; Zompa, E. A.; Cain, L.; Morshed, T.; Hulsebosch, C. E. (1997). Culture, expansion, and transplantation of human fetal neural progenitor cells. *Transplant Proc*, 29, 2040-2041.

[175] Feldmann, R. E., Jr; Bieback, K.; Maurer, M. H.; Kalenka, A.; Bürgers, H. F.; Gross, B.; Hunzinger, C.; Klüter, H.; Kuschinsky, W.; Eichler, H. (2005). Stem cell proteomes: A profile of human mesenchymal stem cells derived from umbilical cord blood. *Electrophoresis*, 26, 2749-2758.

[176] Wagner W, Feldmann RE Jr, Seckinger A, Maurer MH, Wein F, Blake J, Krause U, Kalenka A, Bürgers HF, Saffrich R, Wuchter P, Kuschinsky W, Ho AD (2006). The heterogeneity of human mesenchymal stem cell preparations - evidence from simultaneous analysis of proteomes and transcriptomes. *Exp Hematol*, 34, 536-548.

In: Neural Stem Cell Research
Editor: Eric V. Grier, pp. 77-97

ISBN: 1-59454-846-3
© 2006 Nova Science Publishers, Inc.

Chapter 4

TO KNOW NEURAL STEM PROPERTIES FROM DISEASED BRAINS: A CRITICAL STEP FOR BRAIN REPAIR

M. Fernández, M. Paradisi, L. Giardino and L. Calzà*

Animal Stem Cell Laboratory (ASC-Lab), Department of Veterinary Morphophysiology and Animal Production (DIMORFIPA), University of Bologna, Ozzano Emilia, Italy

Abstract

Neural Stem Cell (NSC) research has given light to unknown brain plasticity and potential repair capacities. The understanding of fundamental NSC's properties, resulting from the interaction between intrinsic genetic properties and extrinsic signalling factors, has been possible also thanks to the isolation of these cells from embryonic and adult central nervous system (CNS). Many studies have pointed to the possibility of using these NSCs for cellular therapy and for replacing lost and/or damaged cells by direct grafting after having manipulated them to differentiate into specific neural cell types. Nevertheless, not much information about the properties of NSCs from diseased brains exits. We have standardized isolation, expansion and lineage analysis protocols, for the study of neurospheres and derived cell in adult brain rats in order to investigate possible effects of different experimental diseases and pharmacological treatments on NSCs biological properties. In particular, we have studied adult subventricular zone (SVZ) NSCs and oligodendrocyte precursor cells (OPCs), both *in vivo* and *in vitro*, in terms of proliferation and differentiation in the experimental allergic encephalomyelitis model (EAE, the most used animal model for multiple sclerosis -MS-), induced in rats. The number of primary neurospheres generated from the subventricular zone (SVZ) was higher in EAE compared to control animals. Due to the key role played by thyroid hormone (TH) in oligodendrocyte lineage induction through cell cycle regulation, we also tested the *in vivo* effect of TH on neurospheres generation. TH treatment induced a

---

* Correspondence: M. Fernández , ASC-Lab, DIMORFIPA, Università di Bologna, Via Tolara di Sopra 50, 40064 Ozzano dell'Emilia, ITALY, Phone: +39-051-2097354, Fax: +39-051-2097953, Email:mfernandez@vet.unibo.it

significant decrease in the number of secondary-generated neurospheres. These results support once more the hypothesis that TH participates in cell-cycle exit mechanisms also in adult NSCs. In conclusion, the study of endogenous NSCs properties in pathological brains offers a unique opportunity to explore the *milieu* that regulate endogenous stem cells and that eventually will be encountered by transplanted cells.

Neural stem cells (NSCs) research has been characterized by an extraordinary expansion over the past few years also in view of new possible therapies for neurodegenerative diseases. The use of neural stem-based cell therapy to overcome the scarce potential repair capacity of an injured/diseased brain constitutes one of the more responsible cues that NSCs's research has to deal with. Many studies have focused on the use of NSCs for grafting specific neural cell types into effected areas, in a great number of animal models of neurodegenerative diseases such as Alzheimer disease's (AD) (Jin et al., 2004), Parkinson disease's (PD) (Sanchez-Pernaute et al., 2005; Sorensen et al., 2005), multiple sclerosis (MS) (Pluchino et al., 2003), spinal cord injury (Okano et al., 2002) and stroke (Haas et al., 2005).

In order to unveil the proliferative and differentiative potential of NSCs and their use for cell replacement therapeutic purposes, it is of extreme importance: i) to identify genes responsible for proliferation and/or differentiation regulation of NSCs and to know how they act; ii) to understand the mechanisms that regulate NSCs biological and physiological functions; iii) to study key molecules capable of enhancing the potential of endogenous NSCs to proliferate and differentiate into specific cell phenotypes to achieve structural and functional brain repair. In order to pursue these goals, *in vivo* and *in vitro* models are being used so far. Although *in vivo* models reflect in a more realistic fashion the environment of a diseased brain, due to the complexity of the mechanisms underlying neurodegenerative diseases, simplified *in vitro* approaches are often useful to investigate many fundamental biological processes that take part in these pathologies.

In our recent work, we have attempted to at least partially overcome limitations intrinsic to both *in vivo* and *in vitro* approaches for NSCs understanding, focusing on the *in vitro* study of properties of neurospheres generated from brains of rats affected by experimental pathologies and pharmacologically treated. "Neurospheres" are heterogeneous aggregates of cells, also including NSCs, which can be obtained and expanded from the subventricular zone in the forebrain of adult animals (Pevny and Rao, 2003). We focused in particular on the possible role of endogenous NSCs and oligodendrocyte precursors in the re-myelination capability of the mature central nervous system (CNS). It is in fact well known that remyelination is possibly the only true, robust repair capability of the mature CNS, due to the large number of oligodendrocyte precursor cells (OPCs) which are widely disseminated in the white and grey matter (Chen et al., 2002). However, for unknown reason, this capability is lost or defective in a percentage of patients affected by MS, the most diffuse demyelinating disease (Lubetzki et al., 2005), thus leading to the axonal and neuronal damage which is responsible for chronic disabilities (Bruck and Stadelmann, 2005; D'Intino et al., 2005). Our previous *in vivo* work has demonstrated that NSCs in the SVZ are highly susceptible to the microenvironmental conditions observed in the inflammatory phase of the inflammatory demyelinating disease experimental allergic encephalomyelitis (EAE), which is the most widely used model for MS (Calzà et al., 1998, 2004), whereas other lesions, which includes a low inflammatory response, inhibits rather than stimulates proliferation rate in the SVZ (Calzà et al., 2004). We have also proved that the *in vivo* administration of thyroid hormone

(TH), which is the key signal for oligodendrocyte generation during CNS development, regulates cell proliferation in the SVZ and favours oligodendrocyte generation and maturation (Calzà et al., 2002; Fernández et al., 2004; Calzà et al., 2005). We have proved that EAE induces extensive proliferation of OPCs (NG2-, A2B5- PDGF alfa R-expressing cells) and that administration of TH is able to promote faster and complete myelination. Moreover, expression of cell cycle-associated markers in NSCs in the SVZ, which also proliferate actively in the acute phase of EAE (e.g. under inflammatory stimuli), significantly decreases in EAE rats treated with TH during a precise time-window corresponding to intense proliferation.

We have contributed as well to the hypothesis that oligodendrocyte development and myelination are under TH control not only during development, but also in the adult life, possibly affecting re-myelination capability of the mature CNS (Fernández et al., 2004).

In this paper we present the protocols that we routinely use in the lab for standardization and quantification of neurosphere production from the adult rat brain, for characterization of derived cells and application on diseased brains. All the materials used and the procedures followed have been described in great detail in Appendix 1 and Appendix 2, respectively, in this chapter.

Characterization of Neurospheres and Derived Cells from Adult Rat Brain

NSCs obtained from the SVZ of adult rat brains are able to proliferate and form cell clusters or "neurospheres" when cultivated in suspension in the presence of mitogens, such as epidermal- (EGF) and basic fibroblast growth factor (bFGF) (Reynolds and Weiss, 1996). Neurospheres are aggregates of heterogeneous cells also containing NSCs, which can be obtained from different brain regions, and particularly from the SVZ, the region immediately beneath the lateral ventricle in the forebrain. According to the pioneer work from Alvarez-Buylla lab, we know that this area contains different cell populations (Alvarez-Buylla and Lim, 2004) that they have called A, B and C. Type B cells are astrocytes identified as the SVZ "stem cell" and the cells that constitute the so called "niche". C cells are rapidly dividing, transit-amplifying cells derived from the B cells. C cells give rise to A cells, neuroblasts that migrate to the olfactory bulb where they become local interneurons. This area can be rapidly dissected, cells finely dissociated and cultured in suspension. Along the days *in vitro*, the number of cells inside the aggregates increased and neurospheres grow in size.

Cells with no proliferative capacity are not able to generate cell clusters. These cells can be observed in the cultures as single cells or even in groups of 2-3 cells at the beginning of the *in vitro* period (1-3 DIV) but they are not potential neurospheres. At 7 DIV, the number of neurospheres generated from NSCs cultured without mitogens is significantly smaller compared with EGF/bFGF-treated cultures (Fig. 1B). When studying *in vitro* cell proliferation, not only the number of generated neurospheres but also their size should be considerate. As previously mentioned, the higher neurosphere mean diameter value, the higher number of cells inside it. Along the days in culture neurospheres mean diameter value shift from score 1 (including cell cluster having diameter ranging from 1 to 50 μm) to score 2 (50-100 μm) and 3 (≥100 μm) (Fig. 1D). On the other hand, proliferation and cell

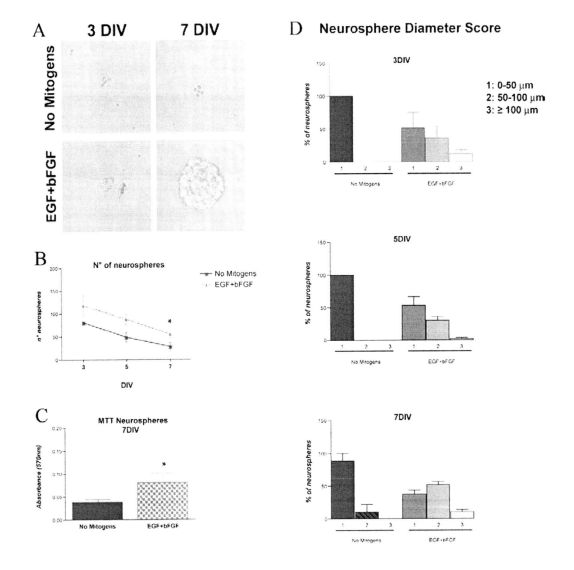

Fig. 1. Cell proliferation and viability. A. Representative images of neurospheres at 3 and 7 DIV, from no mitogens and EGF/bFGF-treated groups. Magnification 20x. B. The number of primary generated neurospheres (no mitogens and EGF/bFGF-treated) at different days in culture is represented in the graph. C. MTT assay performed to no mitogens and EGF/bFGF-treated neurospheres at 7 DIV. Absorbance lecture at 570nm is represented in the graph. D. Diameter score of neurospheres at 3-5 and 7 DIV.

survival can be studied by the MTT method, which gives quantitative information about living cells by measuring the activity of mitochondrial succinate dehydrogenase enzymes. At 7 DIV the absorbance values obtained from EGF/bFGF-treated neurospheres are significantly higher than values obtained from no mitogens group (Fig. 1C), matching quantification of morphological analysis.

As already mentioned, neurospheres are aggregates of heterogeneous cells which can be characterized for the expression of specific antigens, e.g. by flow cytometry (Parker et al., 2005; Kim and Morshead, 2003), gene-chip microarray (Parker et al., 2005), antibody microarray (Ko et al., 2005a, b), immunocytochemistry (Ko et al., 2005b; Moeller and Dimitrijevich, 2004). Immunocytochemistry has the great advantage to leave neurospheres intact, so that distribution of different markers in the periphery *versus* the core of the neurosphere can be described. A great number of both surface and intracellular antigens have been proposed as "specific" for certain lineage and differentiation stage, and the list of "crucial" signalling molecules for NSCs regulation is daily growing. Figure 2 shows images of secondary generated neurospheres at 7 days-in-vitro (DIV) immunoreactive (IR) for nestin, MCM2 (minichromosome maintenance type-2), GFAP (glial fibrillary acidic protein) and doublecortin (DCX) (panels A, B, C and D, respectively), counter-stained with the specific nuclear colorant Hoechst 33258. Nestin-immunoreactivity can be observed in almost all the cells composing the neurosphere, revealing the undifferentiated state of these neuroectodermal cells. Nestin is in fact an intermediate filament protein expressed in dividing cells during the early stages of development in the CNS, PNS and in myogenic and other tissues (Michalczyk and Ziman, 2005). Minichromosome maintenance family of proteins (MCM2 to MCM7) are regulators that act to ensure DNA replication to occurs only once in the cell cycle (Masai and Arai, 2002). The expression of these proteins increases during cell growth, peaking at G1 to S cell cycle phase. MCM2-immunoreactivity indicates cells in proliferative state (Fig. 2 B). As illustrated in Fig. 2B, MCM2-expressing cells, as showed by the white nuclei (arrows) due to the overlap of the IR-signal (green) and the nuclear staining (blue), represent a percentage of the total number of cells. Astrocyte-lineage cells are identified by GFAP antibody. A great number of neurosphere cells GFAP positive can be observed, showing the typical morphology of astrocytes (Fig. 2 C). The microtubule binding protein doublecortin (DCX) is a marker for adult neurogenesis (Friocourt et al., 2003). Its expression is induced in neuronal progenitors individualizing in this way neural lineage, only while they are being generated. DCX-positive cells with not defined processes show the morphology of migrating neuronal precursor cells. Positive DCX elements can be identified in the core of the neurospheres and also in some cell that have started to migrate away from the cluster (Fig. 2 D).

Rat, murine and human neurospheres have been demonstrated to be spontaneously multipotent (e.g. capable of generating neurons, astrocytes and oligodendrocytes). A great effort has been devoted to the development of culture conditions able to increase either neural or oligodendroglial lineage. We have instead studied spontaneous lineage from neurospheres derived from diseased and/or treated brains. When neurospheres find an appropriate substratum they attach and migrate away from the core of the cluster, starting to differentiate in any of the known neural lineage cell type (neurons, astrocytes or oligodendrocytes). After neurospheres splitting, obtained cells can be cultured on appropriate substrates to make them attach and differentiate in a medium without mitogens. Cells will show a more differentiated status with the days in culture. As in the case of neurospheres, differentiated cells can be characterized by protein- and messenger RNA-based techniques, which are used to study the expression of different proteins and genes, markers of cell types in different state of their lineage. Cells obtained from neurospheres and cultured in a medium without mitogens for 7 days have been processed for immunocytochemical detection of specific markers and for the

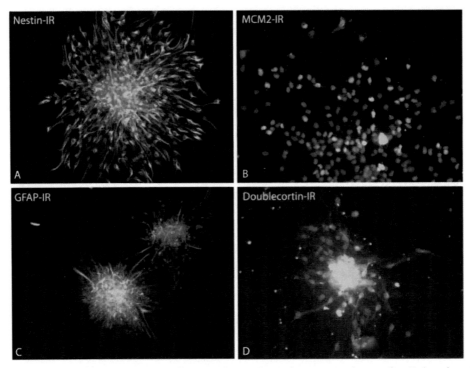

Fig. 2. Immunocytochemical staining of neurospheres. Secondary neurospheres after 7 days in culture were attached to coated coverslips and processed for immunocytochemistry after 24h. Cells exhibiting nestin (A), MCM2 (B), GFAP (C), or doublecortin (D) immunoreactivity are showed. In all the cases counterstaining with Hoechst 33258 was performed. Magnification 20x.

morphological analysis (Fig. 3). Double and triple stainings can be also applied, in order to calculate the percentage of cells in each lineage. Cells double stained with nestin/MCM2 and counterstained with Hoechst 33258 are showed in Fig. 3 A-D. Positive-nestin/MCM2 cells can be observed, however not all the cells are immunoreactive for both antigens. In fact some cells identified by Hoechst (nucleus) do not present nestin- nor MCM2-immunoreactivity (cells into the circle). Some cells are nestin-positive/MCM2-negative. On the contrary, nestin-negative/MCM2-positive cells can be observed (Fig. 3 B-C-D). NG2 is an integral membrane chondroitin sulfate proteoglycan present in the surfaces of some developing and mature central nervous system cells that have properties of oligodendrocyte precursor cells (Reynolds et al., 2002). NG2-IR cells shows the typical OPCs morphology, characterized by a small cell body, radial, finely branched and short elongation and proliferating activity. Many NG2-positive/MCM2-positive cells can be observed (Fig. 3 F,H). Not all the cells are NG2-positive (Fig. 3E) and in the same way not all the cells are MCM2 immunoreactive (Fig. 3H). "Rip"-positive cells, which are small, short and distally branched elongation, have been identified in our cultures of differentiated primary NSCs (Fig. 3L), indicating the presence of mature oligodendrocytes (Friedman et al., 1989). Glial fibrillar acidic protein-positive cells showing the classical morphology of astrocytes are included in Fig. 3M. Finally, cells exhibiting neuronal lineage have been also identified by Tuj1 and NF 68KDa (neurofilament 68KDa) antibodies (Fig. 3 I,N). Tuj1 (class III beta-tubulin) is a marker of neurons in the central and

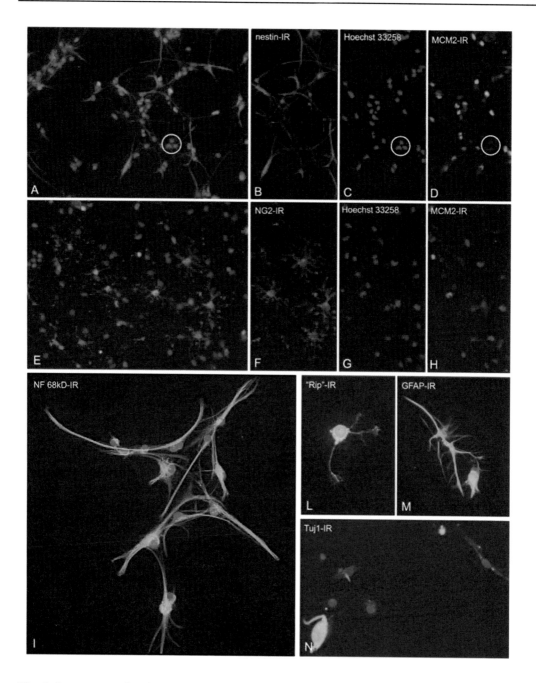

Fig. 3. Immunocytochemical characterization of cells derived from neurospheres. Cell obtained from neurosphere splitting and cultured on coated coverslips in a medium without mitogenes for 7 days were studied by immunocytochemistry. Nestin/MCM2- as well as NG2/MCM2-doublestaining was performed. A: cells nestin-positive counterstained with Hoechst 33258; B, C, D: nestin-, Hoechst-, MCM2-stained cells, respectively. Magnification 20x. E: NG2/MCM2-doublestained cells; F, G, H: NG2-, Hoechst-, MCM2-stained cells. Neuronal lineage markers, NF 68 KDa and Tuj1, are expressed by differentiated cells (I and N, respectively). Cells positive for glial lineage antigen markers such as Rip (oligodendroglial) (L) and GFAP (astroglial) (L) are also present in our primary cultures of NSCs. Panel I has been generated by using a deconvolution program.

peripheral nervous systems from the early stage of neural differentiation (Katsetos et al., 2003). Neurofilaments (NFs) (representative class of intermediate filaments that constitute a major part of the cellular cytoskeleton), are excellent markers for neurons and they can be also expressed by some cells of neural crest origin (Petzold, 2005). Based of this antigen-expression study we can argue that in our primary cultures of differentiated cells derived from adult neurospheres are present both, NSCs and progenitors, which are still proliferating but already committed to a given cell fate. Cells expressing antigens markers of more mature lineage stage, NF- and "Rip"-positive cells for instance, have been also observed. In order to perform a quantitative characterization, cells positive for different markers (undifferentiated cells, proliferating cells, neuronal, astroglial and oligodendroglial lineage at different maturation stages) have been counted and expressed in percentage of total number of cells. Results are presented in Table I. This type of analysis can be also carried out in cell derived from neurospheres generated from diseased brain, in order to analyze the possible effect of the disease on the intrinsic properties of these cells.

Table I. Immunocytochemistry characterization of cells derived from neurospheres. Cells obtained from 7 DIV neurosphere (primary and secondary) splitting and cultured in a medium without mitogens for another 7 days have been processed for immunocytochemistry. Cells positive for the different antibodies used have been counted and referred to the total number of cells (Hoechst 33258 stained) as a percentage. Coexistence of different markers has not been quantified. **Abbreviations not mentioned in the text**: EGFr, epidermal growth factor receptor; MAP2, microtubule-associated protein; A2B5, marker for immature OPCs

Lineage	Antibody	Primary Neurospheres % Positive Cells	Secondary Neurospheres % Positive Cells
Undifferentiated	Nestin	37	17.2
	EGFr	60.8	29.5
Proliferation	MCM2	60	37.7
Neuronal	TuJ1	12.3	7.6
	MAP2	34.3	32.7
Astroglial	GFAP	28	3.5
Oligodendroglial	A2B5	41.1	14.9
	NG2	29.5	21.6
	Rip	25.7	7.2

Neurospheres from EAE Brain

As previously mentioned, one of our aims is to apply the knowledge obtained from the adult rat brain NSCs on diseased brains, in particular in demyelinating diseased brains, using for that the EAE-induced animal model. We have previously reported from *in vivo* studies that EAE induces proliferation in the SVZ (Calzà et al., 1998; Picard-Reira et al., 2002) and that TH administration in a precise time-window can decrease proliferation, induce oligodendrocyte lineage (Calzà et al., 2002), favour remyelination and modify the clinical out-come of ill animals (Fernández et al., 2004). In this case, we have studied the *in vitro* proliferation rate of NSCs obtained from the SVZ of EAE-induced animals by analyzing: i) the number of generated primary and secondary neurospheres; ii) neurosphere mean diameter. After 7 days in culture, primary and secondary neurospheres generated from control, EAE and EAE+T4 groups of animals were counted and photographed. Results are reported in Fig. 4.

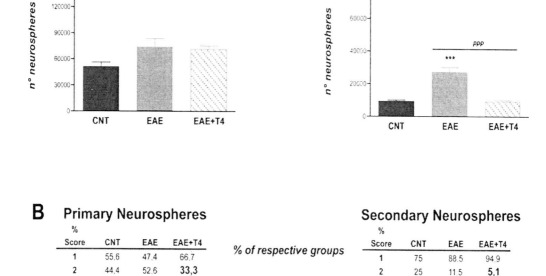

Fig. 4. In vitro proliferation rate of EAE NSCs. A. Number of primary and secondary generated neurospheres from control, EAE and EAE+T4 groups of animals after 7 days in culture. The number of secondary neurospheres from EAE animals was significantly higher than in the control group; T4 treatment inducted a significant decrease in the number of secondary neurospheres. Statistical analysis was performed by one-way ANOVA and Tukey's multiple comparison post-test, *** $P<0.001$, ppp $P<0.001$. Results are shoe as mean ± SEM of two different cultures performed. B. Mean diameter values of primary and secondary generated neurospheres were obtained with Image Pro-Plus software. Neurospheres were classified in the base of their mean diameter; the number of neurospheres obtained from control animals with score 1 or score 2 were considered as 100%; the number of neurospheres from EAE and EAE+T4-treated animals with diameter score 1 or 2 was referred to control group. EAE animals generated a higher number of score 2 primary neurospheres, meanwhile EAE+T4 treated animals generated a smaller number of score 2 secondary neurospheres.

The number of primary generated neurospheres from EAE- and EAE+T4-animals was higher comparing with control animals, however these differences were not significant. On the contrary, the number of secondary neurospheres from EAE animals was significantly higher than control group; T4 treatment induced a decrease of 66 % in the number of secondary neurospheres obtained from EAE animals.

Neurospheres were classified in the base of their mean diameter, which was calculated as described in Appendix 2 (section 2.4). The number of neurospheres obtained from control animals, score 1 and score 2, were considered as 100%. Proliferation rate of NSCs from the SVZ of EAE animals is increased as bigger primary neurospheres and a significant higher number of secondary neurospheres have been generated. T4 treatment provoked a decrease in the proliferation rate as a significantly lower number of secondary neurospheres and a lower number of obtained score 2 neurospheres have revealed.

Future Directions

PCR technology is widely used to quantify DNA because the amplification of the target sequence allows for greater sensitivity of detection than could be achieved with any other method. Real-time fluorescence-based quantitative PCR (QPCR) represents a revolutionary technique that has overcome the problems of conventional PCR. It has been established as the reference technology for the quantification of nucleic acids because of its high precision and sensitivity, offering an immense choice of protocols and chemistries. Gene expression instrument and reaction conditions, as well as the right combination of fluorophores to label probes. The more important advantage of multiplex PCR reactions is the reduced sample requirement, which is especially important when sample material is scarce, as in the case of NSCs cultivated from the SVZ of adult rat brains. Nestin, that constitutes a very useful marker for NSC's study, and many other genes that are useful markers for proliferation or for different fates in the lineage of committed cells can be studied with high precision using this technique. Panels D, E and F in Fig. 5 show amplification plot, dissociation curve and standard curve, respectively, obtained from nestin QPCR performed using the SYBR Green I chemistry after the optimisation of the assay.

Laser microdissection is a high technology method that allows isolation of small areas or single cells from histological preparations (sections) or from culture dish, respectively, in order to be used for further analysis. Only desiderated cells are cut out from the preparation under microscopic view, with high precision. Since the cut is followed without mechanical contact, laser capture microdissection (LCM) permits the isolation of specific cell types for subsequent cell tissue culture as well as for molecular (DNA, RNA) and protein analysis. Figure 5 (A, B and C) shows the image of a tolouidine blue stained section (panel A), which has been used for the isolation of the SVZ by LCM after designing the area to cut (panel B). The section after the capture of the SVZ is showed in panel C.

LCM and subsequent real-time QPCR in selected areas of tissue section or in single cells from a either sections or culture dish can help us to understand the neurobiology as well as the molecular mechanism that take part in NSCs and progenitors regulation from both, health and diseased brain, with a very high cellular specificity. This is a crucial point in further understanding the biology of adult NSCs and derived cells, also in view of stem-based cell therapy.

Appendix 1: Materials

1.1. Animals
- Adult male Sprague-Dawley rats (250-400 g body weight)
- Adult female Lewis rats (150-175 g body weight)
- Adult female Dark-Agouti rats (150-175 g body weight)

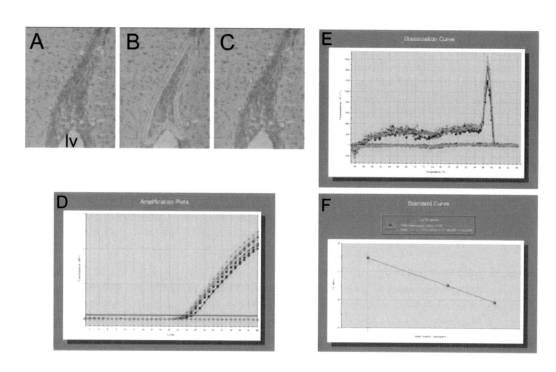

Fig. 5. Laser capture microdissection + QPCR: foremost techniques for NSCs research. The SVZ of adult rat can be specifically isolated thanks to the laser capture microdissection technique. Panels A, B and C show a tolouidine blue stained section, designed area to cut and the section after the capture of the SVZ, respectively. Panels D, E and F show amplification plot, dissociation curve and standard curve, respectively, obtained from nestin QPCR performed using the quantification, expression profiling, validation of microarray data and others are research applications of QPCR. Moreover, multiplex PCR assay makes possible the simultaneous amplification of up to four genes in a single reaction tube when using the appropriate SYBR Green I chemistry after the optimisation of the assay. The efficiency of the PCR is 102% (F). Nestin primers have been designer with *Beacon Designer 4.0* software, for the amplification of a 262 bp fragment.

1.2. Models Preparation (EAE)
- Adult female Lewis or Dark-Agouti rats
- Guinea pig spinal cord tissue
- Complete Freund's adjuvant (Sigma, cat. n° F5881)
- Heat-inactivated *Mycobacterium* (Difco H37Ra, cat. n° 231141)
- Bidistilated water bbH$_2$O
- Sterile physiologic solution

- Homogenator (Ultra Turrax, IKA-WERKE, Germany)

1.3. Primary NSC Culture Preparation

- Standard tissue culture and dissection equipment.
- Enzymes: Trypsin (Sigma, cat. n°. T4665), Hyaluronidase (Sigma, cat. n°. H3884), Deoxyribonuclease (Sigma, cat. n°. D4527), Trypsin/EDTA solution (Sigma, cat. n°. 35400-019).
- Serum-free complete growth medium: DMEM (Dulbecco's Modified Eagle Medium) / F12 (1:1) GLUTAMAX I (Gibco/BRL, cat. n°. 31331-028), B27 supplement (Gibco/BRL, cat. n°. 12587-010), N-2 (Gibco/BRL, cat. n°. 17502-048), 8 mM HEPES (Gibco/BRL, cat. n°. 15630-056), 100 U/mL penicillin, 100 µg/mL streptomycin (Sigma, cat. n°. 15140-122).
- Mitogens: EGF (Gibco/BRL, cat. n°.13247-051), bFGF (10ng/ml) (Euro-Clon, cat. n°. PPH090050).
- HBSS (without Ca2+/Mg2+) (Gibco/BRL, cat. n°. 14170-088), EBSS (Gibco/BRL, cat. n°. 24010-043), 1M HEPES (Gibco/BRL).
- BSA (Bovine Serum Albumin) (Sigma, cat. n°. A4503), Sucrose (Sigma, cat. n°. S1888), D-Glucose (Sigma, cat. n°. G8769).
- Poly-L-lysine (Sigma, cat. n°. P1524).
- Poly-L-ornithine (Sigma, cat. n°. P4957).
- Laminin (Sigma, cat. n°. L2020).
- 0,22µm and 70µm sterile filters (Falcon).

1.4. Immunocytochemistry

- Primary antibodies: anti-Nestin (mouse monoclonal antibody, PharMingen, CA), 1:500; anti EGF-r (sheep polyclonal, Upstate), 1:75; anti-MCM-2 (goat polyclonal, Chemicon), 1:150; anti-doublecortin (goat polyclonal, Santa Cruz), 1:150; anti-β-tubulin (mouse monoclonal, β III isoform, R & D systems) 1:1000; anti-NF (rabbit polyclonal, Chemicon), 1:100; anti-MAP-2 (rabbit polyclonal, Chemicon); anti-A2B5 (mouse monoclonal MAB312R, Chemicon) 1:500; anti-NG2 chondroitin sulphate proteoglycan (rabbit polyclonal, Chemicon) 1:250; anti-oligodendrocyte "Rip" (MAB 1580 mouse monoclonal, clone "RIP", Chemicon International, Inc), 1:2500 ; anti MBP (rabbit polyclonal, DAKO, Carpinteria) 1:200; anti-GFAP (mouse monoclonal, clone G-A-5, Chemicon International, Inc), 1:100. See Table II bellow.
- Fluorescent secondary antibodies (Donkey-FITC or Donkey-RRX conjugated, Jackson).
- Phosphate buffered saline (PBS)
- 0.2M Sørensen phosphate buffer: Prepare stock solutions A (0.2 M NaH_2PO_4) and B (0.2 M Na_2HPO_4). Mix 280 ml of Solution A and 720 ml of Solution B.
- 4% Paraformaldehyde in 0.1M Sørensen phosphate buffer: prepare an 8% paraformaldehyde solution in ddH_2O, so stir constantly, warm to 50-55°C (don't exceed 58°C) and add 2N NaOH till all paraphormaldehyde has been dissolved. Filter the solution through filter paper, add an equal volume of 0.2M Sörensen buffer, adjust pH to 7.4 and conserve at 4°C.
- Triton X-100 (Merk, cat. n°. K32942203 417).
- Phenylendiamine mounting solution: 0.1% 1,4-phenylendiamine (Sigma, cat. n°.), 50% glycerine (Sigma, cat. n°. G5150), carbonate/bicarbonate buffer pH 8.6.

- Normal serum donkey
- Hoechst 33258 (Sigma, cat. n°. 23491-45-4)

1.5. Microscopy

- Olympus IX70 inverted microscope + Olympus digital camera
- Olympus Provis + F-View camera and SoftImagingSystem (SIS, Munster, Germany). Filters: WG2 (ex 510-550nm, DM 570, emission 590nm), NU2 (ex 360-370nm, DM 400, emission 420nm), NIBA2 (ex 470-490, DM 505, emission 510-550nm),

Table II. Antibodies routinely used for neurospheres and derived cells immunocytochemistry

Antibody	Supplier	Code	Dilution
A2B5	Chemicon	MAB312R	1:1000
BrdU	Immunological Direct	OBT0030	1:100
CNPase	Chemicon	MAB326R	1:250
Doublecortin	SantaCruz	sc-8066	1:150
EGFr	UpState	06-129	1:75
GFAP	Chemicon	MAB3402	1:100
MAP2	Chemicon	MAB3418	1:350
MCM2	SantaCruz	sc-9839	1:150
Musashi	Chemicon	AB5977	1:250
Nestin	Pharmingen	556309	1:500
NF 68KD	Chemicon	AB1983	1:100
NG2	Chemicon	AB5320	1:250
O4	Chemicon	MAB345	1:200
PSA-NCAM	Pharmingen	556325	1:300
Rip	Chemicon	MAB1580	1:2500
Tuj1	R&D System	MAB1195	1:1000

- Olympus FluoView 500 laser scan confocal microscope on Olympus IX81 inverted microscope

1.6. MTT assay

- MTT solution (5mg/ml): dissolve MTT (Sigma, cat. n°. M5655) in Opti-MEM (without phenol red) (Gibco/BRL, cat. n°. 11058-021). Filter sterilize keeping the solution protected from the light at 4°C.
- Isopropanol (Merk cat. n°. I044294 228)
- 1M HCl (Merk, cat. n°. K28466517 046)
- Microplate reader (Model 680 Microplate Reader, Bio-Rad)

1.7. mRNA isolation and DNase treatment
- mRNA isolation Kit (Roche Molecular Biochemical's cat. n°. 1 741 985)
- RNase-DNase-free H_2O (dd H_2O DEP-C treated) (DEP-C Sigma, cat. n° D5758)
- Deoxyribonuclease I ribonuclease-free (DNase I) (Fermentas, Life Sciences cat. n°. EN0521)
- Dithiothreitol (DTT) 0,1M (Sigma, cat. n° D9779)
- Ribonuclease inhibitor (RNase) 40 U/µl (Fermentas, Life Sciences cat. n°. EO 0381)
- Molecular biology grade bbH_2O

1.8. Reverse Transcription
- mRNA
- 5x First Strand Buffer (Fermentas Life Sciences, cat. n°. EP 0441)
- Moloney-Murine Leukaemia Virus (M-MuLV) reverse transcriptase (RT) enzyme (Fermentas Life Sciences, cat. n°. EP 0441).
- 100 mM deoxynucleoside triphosphate d(NTP)s (Sigma, cat. n°. DNTP-100)
- 1mM p(dN)$_6$ random primers (Roche Molecular Biochemicals, cat. n°. 1 034 731)

1.9. Real-time Polymerase Chain Reaction (PCR)
- cDNA (retrotranscribed mRNA)
- 2X Brilliant SYBR Green QPCR Master Mix (Stratagene, cat. n°. 600458)
- Beacon Designer 4.0 software
- Nestin primers (MWG-Biotech AG)

    Upstream: 5'-GGAGTGTCGCTTAGAGGTGC-3'

    Downstream: 5'-CAGCAGAGTCCTGTATGTAGCC-3'
- Mx3005P Real-Time PCR system (Stratagene)

1.10. Laser Microdissection
- Cryostat system (1720 Kryostat, Leitz)
- Vibratome 800, McIIwain Tissue Chopper (Ted Pella Inc.)
- Tolouidine Blue solution (196 mM acetic acid, 4 mM sodium acetate, 27 mM Toluidine Blue).
- SLµCut Microdissection system (Molecular Machines & Industries) on Nikon Eclipse TE2000S
- Laser microdissection slides / chambers
- Sterile reaction tubes for laser microdissection

Appendix 2: Methods

2.1. Experimental allergic encephalomyelitis (EAE) induction.
Animal care and treatments were in accordance with European Community Council Directives of November 24, 1986 (86/609/EEC) and approved by our intramural committee and Ministero Istruzione, Università e Ricerca, in compliance with the guidelines published in the National Institutes of Health Guide for the Care and Use of Laboratory Animals.

1. Prepare an emulsion by homogenising with guinea pig spinal cord tissue (0.15 g/ml), complete Freund's adjuvant (50% vol/vol) and heat-inactivated *Mycobacterium* (Difco H37Ra) (5 mg/ml). Inject 100µl in hindlimb footpads.
2. Check daily the advancement of the EAE by evaluating the evolution of clinic parameters which indicate animals' state of health and give right score from 0 to

5 depending on observed symptoms: 0- no symptoms; 1- limp tail; 2- hindlimb weakness; 3- hindlimb paralysis; 4- quadriplegia; 5- severe paralysis and incontinence.

2.2. Primary NSCs cultures

The following protocol is based in the protocol described by Clarke et al., (2000) which has been properly changed and adapted to our conditions.

1. Remove the brain and put in cold sterilized PBS

The procedure is now followed under laminar flow hood.

2. Make first a coronal cut frontal to the hypothalamus area discarding the caudal part of brain. Then make a sagittal cut in order to separate the two hemispheres. Take off areas surrounding lateral ventricles and acutely dissect the anterior portion of the lateral wall's lateral ventricle (SVZ) from both brain hemispheres.
3. Dissociate tissue, first enzymatically in a solution containing 1.3 mg/mL trypsin, 0.7 mg/mL hyaluronidase, 1000U deoxyribonuclease, 5.4 mg/mL D-Glucose in HBSS, incubating at 37°C for 20 min, and then mechanically using a fire-polished Pasteur pipette.
4. Filter through a nylon mesh filter (70μm).
5. Add a solution of 0.308 g/mL sucrose in HBSS, in order to remove myelin fragments and centrifugate (500xg, 5 min).
6. Wash pellet with a solution of 40 mg/mL BSA, 20 mM HEPES in EBSS pH 7.5, centrifuge and resuspend cell pellet in serum-free culture medium (described above).
7. Seed cells to a density between $3\text{-}5x10^3$ cells/cm^2. Add mitogens (EGF 20ng/mL, bFGF 10ng/ml) to the medium every 48 h. Group of cells with "8" shape can be observed after 1 DIV. Spherical shape and phase-bright outer edges are useful criterion to identify true neurospheres, easily visible after 3-4 DIV.

For the study of *in vitro* cell proliferation, count and photograph primary generated neurospheres after 6-7 days in culture, in order to perform neurosphere number and mean diameter analyses, respectively.

Primary neurospheres can be used for immunocytochemical characterization after having been attached to an appropriate substratum, or for the generation of secondary neurospheres, which can be used for immunocytochemical characterization and/or for the study of differentiated cells, after having been split.

2.3. Neurospheres Splitting

When appropriate, split primary neurospheres to generate secondary neurospheres or to obtain differentiated cells.

1. Spin neurospheres down at 1500 rpm.
2. Incubate with Trypsin/EDTA solution at 37°C for 8 minutes and centrifuge.
3. Pass pellet through a fire-polished Pasteur pipette, add a solution containing 40 mg/mL BSA, 20 mM HEPES in EBSS pH 7.59 and centrifuge again.
4. Resuspend cell pellet in serum-free medium.

For the generation of secondary neurospheres:

5. Seed cells to a density between $3\text{-}5x10^3$ cells/cm^2. Add mitogens (EGF 20ng/mL, bFGF 10ng/ml) to the medium every 48 h.

2.4. Immunocytochemistry

Differentiated cells can be characterized by immunocytochemistry. The commercially available antibodies listed in TABLE I have been used at the indicated dilutions

2.4.1. Neurospheres Immunocytochemistry.

Neurospheres can be characterized by immunocytochemistry by making them to attach to an appropriate substrate.

Prepare plates as follow:

1. Place sterile glass coverslips in 4-well or 24-well plates and treat them with 0.5 ml of poly-L-ornithine (10µg/ml) overnight at RT on the shaker.
2. Wash coverslips with ddH$_2$O
3. Add laminin (10µg/ml) and incubate at 37°C for 2 h.
4. Wash with PBS and keep under laminar flow hood and UV light for at least 3 h in order to let coverslips dry.

Treated plates can be conserved at 4°C for 1 week.

Prepare neurospheres for immunocytochemistry as follow:

1. After 6-7 DIV, count neurospheres and spin them down at 1500 rpm.
2. Take off surnatant (old medium), filter (0.22µm) and keep it.
3. Acutely, resuspend the pellet with a wide tip pipettor in medium.
4. Seed neurospheres to a density between 50-100 neurospheres/well.
5. Place plates in an incubator and let neurospheres to attach at least for 24 h.

Immunocytochemistry procedure:

1. Wash cells with PBS and fix them with 4% paraformaldehyde for 20 min at RT.
2. Wash three times (5 min each) with PBS and incubate with primary antibodies (diluted in PBS / 0.3% Triton X-100 / 1% normal serum donkey / 1% BSA) overnight at 4°C. Antibody dilutions: anti-Nestin 1:500; anti EGF-r 1:75; anti-MCM-2 1:150; anti-doublecortin 1:150; anti-β-tubulin 1:1000; anti-NF 1:100; anti-MAP-2 1:1000; anti-A2B5 1:500; anti-NG2 1:250; anti-oligodendrocyte "Rip" 1:2500; anti MBP 1:200; anti-GFAP, 1:100.
3. Wash cells (3 x 5 min) with PBS and incubated with secondary antibodies diluted 1:100, for 30 min at 37°C.
4. After PBS washing, incubate with Hoechst 33258 nuclear colorant (1 µg/mL in PBS, 0.2% Triton X-100) for 20 min at RT.
5. Wash with PBS and mount coverslips with phenylendiamine.
6. Count cells in at least five different fields of the coverslip using the 20x objective.

2.4.2. Cell immunocytochemistry

For the study of *in vitro* cell differentiation, after neurospheres splitting (section 2.3) make cells attach to the appropriate substratum. Prepare plates as follow:

1. Place sterile glass coverslips in 4-well or 24-well plates and treat them with 0.5 ml of poly-L-lysine (50µg/ml) solution for 1h and 30 min.
2. Wash coverslips with PBS first and with ddH$_2$O then, keeping plates under laminar flow hood with UV light for at least 3 h.
3. Treated plates can be conserved at 4°C for 1 week.

Seed cells onto poly-L-lysine coated plates at the indicated density and grow them in the same medium without adding mitogens in order to let them differentiate.

The procedure for cell immunocytochemistry is the same that for neurospheres immunocytochemistry Described Above (Section 2.2.1).

2.5. Images And Figure generation

All presented images are generated by acquisition through digital cameras. Double and triple staining are produced by single channel acquisition and color merge using the SIS software. Figures were generated by Photoshop.

2.6. Neurospheres Analysis Diameter

In vitro cell proliferation was study by neurosphere number and mean diameter analyses. Images of photographed neurospheres were used for the analysis of mean diameter using Image-Pro Plus software. Neurospheres were classified in the base of their mean diameter. Neurospheres with mean diameter value between 0-50 µm were given a score 1; neurospheres with mean diameter value between 50-100 µm were given a score 2; neurospheres with mean diameter value ≥100 µm were given a score 2. Finally the number of neurospheres with score 1, 2 or 3 were counted and obtained numbers were expressed in percentage.

2.7. MTT Neurospheres Assay

MTT is a colorimetric assay for the study of mammalian cell survival and proliferation. Mitochondrial succinate dehydrogenases, present in viable cells, use MTT (3-(4,5-dimethylthiazol-2-yl)-2,5-diphenyl tetrazolium bromide) (yellow dye) as a substrate transforming it into formazan crystals (blue). The intensity of the blue color obtained after dissolving formazan formed crystals (measured with the spectrophotometer) gives quantitative information about present living cells.

1. Centrifuge to pellet neurospheres (500xg, 5 min).
2. Add 50µl of MTT solution to the pellet, transfer to a well plate and let it in the incubator for 2 h avoiding light.
3. Add the same volume (50µl) of MTT solvent mixing well and let for 1 h at RT on the shaker.
4. Measure absorbance at 570nm.

2.8. mRNA isolation - DNase Treatment / Reverse Transcription

1. For mRNA isolation follow manufacturer's instructions
2. Incubate 100 mg of mRNA with 1U/µl of DNase in the presence of 10 mM DTT and 4 U/µl RNase, at 37°C for 30 min
3. Denature DNase by heating at 95°C for 2 min
4. Incubate mRNA (DNase- treated) in the presence of 1x First Strand Buffer, 1 mM of each deoxynucleoside triphosphate d(NTP)s, 50 µM p(dN)$_6$ random primers and 200 U of RT enzyme, at 42°C for 60 min
5. Denature RT enzyme by heating at 70°C for 10 min

2.9. Real-time Polymerase Chain Reaction (PCR)

DNA binding dyes used as an optional QPCR chemistry, SYBR Green I for instance, are cost effective and easy to use. If primer designer and PCR reactions' optimisation are properly performed, SYBR Green I can be used as a valid QPCR chemistry for gene expression analysis. We have set up QPCR conditions for the study of nestin gene expression, using the DNA binding dye SYBR Green I. Nestin upstream and downstream primers have been designed with *Beacon Designer 4.0* software, for the amplification of a 262 bp fragment. Since SYBR Green I- and reference-dye are light sensitive, avoid it whenever possible. After determining optimal primer concentrations for the assay, the performance of the PCR reaction in terms of efficiency, precision and sensitivity has to be tested by using a serial dilution positive control template. Amplification plot, dissociation curve and standard curve obtained from nestin QPCR are presented in Fig. 5 (D, E and F, respectively). The same procedure should be performed for each gene which expression has to be studied.

Prepare PCR reactions as follow:

1. Prepare a mix reaction consisting of: 1X Brilliant SYBR Green QPCR Master Mix, 16 nM reference dye (ROX), primers sense and antisense to a final concentration of 0,4 μM
2. Add the mix reaction to each sample of template cDNAs and mix the components gently avoiding making bubbles as they can interfere with fluorescence detection
3. Place reactions in the instrument and start the run. The follow two-step PCR program has been performed: 1 cycle of 10 min at 95°C; 40 cycles of: 30 sec at 95°C, 30 sec at 60°C
4. Dissociation program followed consisted of: 1 cycle of 1 min at 95°C; gradual heating from 55°C to 95°C

2.10. Microdissection

1. Prepare tissue sections of appropriate thickness on special slides for laser microdissection
2. When required, stain sections with Toluidine Blue solution for 6 min and dehydrate sections after a quick wash with bbH$_2$O
3. Identify the area or cells of interest
4. Under microscope isolate desiderated area or cells using the LCM instrument

Text of General Interest

1. Moody SA (Ed) *Cell Lineage And fate Determination,* Academic Press, 1999
2. Sell S (Ed) *Stem Cells. Handbook*, Humana Press, 2004
3. Turksen K (Ed) *Embryonic Stem Cells. Methods and Protocols*, vol. 185, Humana Press, 2002
4. Zigova T, Sanberg PR, Sanchez-Ramos JR (Eds) *Neural Stem Cells. Methods and Protocols*, vol. 198, Humana Press, 2002

Acknowledgement

This work has been supported by Regione Emilia-Romagna, Department for Productive Activities, PRRIITT project 2004.

References

[1] Alvarez-Buylla A, Lim DA. For the long run: maintaining germinal niches in the adult brain. *Neuron* 41 (2004) 683-6

[2]   Brazel CY, Limke TL, Osborne JK, Miura T, Cai J, Pevny L, Rao MS. Sox2 expression defines a heterogeneous population of neurospheres-forming cells in the adult murine brain. *Aging Cell* 4 (2005) 197-207

[3]   Bruck W, Stadelman C. The spectrum of multiple sclerosis: new lesson from pathology. *Curr Opin Neurol* 18 (2005) 221-4

[4]   Calzà L, Giardino L, Pozza M, Betteli C, Micera A,Aloe L. Proliferation and phenotype regulation in the subventricular zone during experimental allergic encephalomyelitis: in vivo evidence for a NGF role. *Proc Natl Acad Sci USA* 95 (1998) 3209-3214

[5]   Calza L, Fernández M, Giuliani A, Aloe L, Giardino L. Thyroid hormone activates oligodendrocyte precursors and increases a myelin forming protein and NGF content in the spinal cord during experimental allergic encephalomyelitis. *Proc Natl Acad Sci USA*, 99 (2002) 3258-63.

[6]   Calza L, Giuliani A, Fernández M, Pirondi S, D'Intino G, Aloe L, Giardino L. Neural stem cells and cholinergic neurons: regulation by immunolesion and treatment with mitogens, retinoic acid, and nerve growth factor. *Proc Natl Acad Sci USA* 100 (2003) 7325-30.

[7]   Calza L, Fernández M, Giuliani A, Pirondi S, D'Intino G, Manservigi M, De Sordi N, Giardino L. Stem cells and nervous tissue repair: from in vitro to in vivo. *Prog Brain Res.* 146 (2004) 75-91

[8]   Calza L, Fernández M, Giuliani A, D'Intino G, Pirondi S, Sivilia S, Paradisi M, Desordi N, Giardino L. Thyroid hormone and remyelination in adult central nervous system: a lesson from an inflammatory-demyelinating disease. *Brain Res Brain Res Rev* 48 (2005) 339-46

[9]   Chen ZJ, Negra M, Levine A, Ughrin Y, Levine JM. Oligodendrocyte precursor cells: reactive cells that inhibit axon growth and regeneration. *J Neurocytol* 31 (2002) 481-95.

[10]   D'Intino G, Paradisi M, Fernández M, Giuliani A, Aloe L, Giardino L, Calza L. Cognitive deficit associated with cholinergic and nerve growth factor down-regulation in experimental allergic encephalomyelitis in rats. *Proc Natl Acad Sci USA* 22 (2005) 3070-5

[11]   Fernández M, Giuliani A, Pirondi S, D'Intino G, Giardino L, Aloe L, Levi-Montalcini R, Calza L. Thyroid hormone administration enhances remyelination in chronic demyelinating inflammatory disease. *Proc Natl Acad Sci USA* 101(2004) 16363-8

[12]   Fernández M, Pirondi S, Manservigi M, Giardino L, Calzà L. Thyroid hormone participates in the regulation of neural stem cells and oligodendrocyte precursor cells in the central nervous system of adult rat. *Eur J Neurosci* 20 (2004) 2059-2070

[13]   Friedman B, Hockfield S, Black JA, Woodruff KA, Waxman SG. In situ demonstration of mature oligodendrocytes and their processes: an immunocytochemical study with a new monoclonal antibody, rip. *Glia* 2 (1989) 380-90.

[14] Friocourt G, Koulakoff A, Chafey P, Boucher D, Fauchereau F, Chelly J, Francis F. Doublecortin functions at the extremities of growing neuronal processes. *Cereb Cortex* 13 (2003) 620-6

[15] Haas S, Weidner N, Winkler J, Adult stem cell therapy in stroke. *Curr Opin Neurol* 18 (2005) 59-64.

[16] Jin K, Galvan V, Xie L, Mao XO, Gorostiza OF, Bredesen DE, Greenberg DA. Enhanced neurogenesis in Alzheimer's disease transgenic (PDGF-APPSw,Ind) mice. *Proc Natl Acad Sci USA* 101 (2004) 13363-7.

[17] Katsetos CD, Herman MM, Mork SJ. Class III beta-tubulin in human development and cancer. *Cell Motil Cytoskeleton* 55 (2003)77-96

[18] Kim M and Morshead CM. Distinct populations of Forebrain Neural Stem and Progenitor Cells Can Be Isolated Using Side-Population Analysis. *J Neurosci* 23 (2003) 10703-10709

[19] Ko KI, Kato K, Iwata H. Antibody microarray for correlating cell phenotype with surface marker. *Biomaterials* 26 (2005a) 687-696

[20] Ko KI, Kato K, Iwata H. Parallel analysis of multiple surface markers expressed on rat neural stem cells using antibody microarrays. *Biomaterials* 26 (2005b) 4882-4891

[21] Lubetzki C, Williams A, Stankoff B. Promoting repair in multiple sclerosis: problems and prospects. *Curr Opin Neurol* 18 (2005) 237-44

[22] Masai H, Arai K. Cdc7 kinase complex: a key regulator in the initiation of DNA replication. *J Cell Physiol* 190 (2002) 287-296

[23] Michalczyk K and Ziman M. Nestin structure and predicted function in cellular cytoskeletal organisation. *Histol Histopathol* 20 (2005) 665-71

[24] Moeller ML, Dimitrijevich SD. A new strategy for analysis of phenotype marker antigens in hollow neurospheres. *J Neurosci Methods* 139 (2004) 43-50

[25] Ogawa Y, Sawamoto K, Miyata T, Miyao S, Watanabe M, Nakamura M, Bregman BS, Koike M, Uchiyama Y, Toyama Y, Okano H. Transplantation of in vitro-expanded fetal neural progenitor cells results in neurogenesis and functional recovery after spinal cord contusion injury in adult rats. *J Neurosci Res* 69 (2002) 925-933

[26] Okano H. Stem cell biology of the central nervous system. *J Neurosci Res* 69 (2002) 698-707

[27] Parker MA, Anderson JK, Corliss DA, Abraria VE, Sidman RL, Park KI, Teng YD, Cotanche DA, Snyder EY. Expression profile of an operationally-defined neural stem cell clone. *Exp Neurol* 194 (2005) 320-332

[28] Petzold A. Neurofilament phosphoforms: surrogate markers for axonal injury, degeneration and loss. *J Neurol Sci* 233 (2005)183-98

[29] Pevny L, Rao MS. The stem-cell menagerie. *Trends Neurosci* 26 (2003) 351-9

[30] Pluchino S, Quattrini A, Brambilla E, Gritti A, Salani G, Dina G, Galli R, Del Carro U, Amadio S, Bergami A, Furlan R, Comi G, Vescovi AL, Martino G. Injection of adult neurospheres induces recovery in a chronic model of multiple sclerosis. *Nature* 422 (2003) 688-94

[31] Reynolds R, Dawson M, Papadopoulos D, Polito A, Di Bello IC, Pham-Dinh D, Levine J. The response of NG2-expressing oligodendrocyte progenitors to demyelination in MOG-EAE and MS. *J Neurocytol* 31 (2002) 523-36

[32] Reynolds BA, Weiss S. Clonal and population analyses demonstrate that an EGF-responsive mammalian embryonic CNS precursor is a stem cell. *Dev Biol* 175 (1996) 1-13

[33] Sanchez-Pernaute R, Studer L, Ferrari D, Perrier A, Lee H, Vinuela A, Isacson O. Long-Term Survival of Dopamine Neurons Derived from Parthenogenetic Primate Embryonic Stem Cells (Cyno-1) After Transplantation. *Stem Cells* 23 (2005) 914-922

[34] Sorensen AT, Thompson L, Kirik D, Bjorklund A, Lindvall O, Kokaia M. Functional properties and synaptic integration of genetically labelled dopaminergic neurons in intrastriatal grafts. *Eur J Neurosci* 21 (2005) 2793-2799

[35] Michalczyk K, Ziman M. Nestin structure and predicted function in cellular cytoskeletal organisation. *Histol Histopathol* (2005) 665-67

In: Neural Stem Cell Research
Editor: Eric V. Grier, pp. 99-114

ISBN: 1-59454-846-3
© 2006 Nova Science Publishers, Inc.

Chapter 5

NEURAL STEM CELLS AND TAURINE

Eulalia Bazán[1], Antonio S. Herranz[1], Diana Reimers[1],
Maria V.T. Lobo[1,2], Carolina Redondo[1], Miguel A. López-
Toledano[1,3], Rafael Gonzalo-Gobernado[1], Maria J. Asensio[1] and
Raquel Alonso[1]*

[1]Servicio de Neurobiología-Investigación, Hospital Ramón y Cajal, Madrid and
[2]Departamento de Biología Celular y Genética, Universidad de Alcalá, Madrid, Spain.
[3]Miguel A. López-Toledano present address: Department of Pathology, Columbia-
Presbyterian Medical Center, Columbia University, 630w, 168th Street.
New York, NY, 10032

Abstract

Taurine is a β-amino acid that serves important functions in mammalian brain development. However, no data are available about its distribution and possible roles in neural precursors from a non-retinal origin. Neural stem cells (NSC) with self-renewal and multilineage potential are an important tool to study the signals involved in the regulation of brain development. The aim of this study was to investigate the role played by taurine during the differentiation of NSC from fetal rat striatum. Taurine content was analyzed in the cultures by HPLC at different times post-plating. Between 2 and 24 hours taurine was detected at a basal value of 7 nmol/mg protein. As cells were maintained in culture, this value increased to reach 40 nmol/mg protein at 10 days post-plating. Taurine immunoreactivity was found in nestin, A2B5, β-tubulin III and O1 positive cells. The addition for 1 to 3 days of 2 mM taurine to recently seeded neurospheres increased its

---

* Corresponding Author: Dr. Eulalia Bazán, Servicio de Neurobiología-Investigación, Hospital Ramón y Cajal, Carretera de Colmenar Km. 9,1, 28034 Madrid, España. Phone: 34-913368384. Fax: 34-913369016. E-mail: eulalia.bazan@hrc.es

intracellular content by 28 fold, and high taurine levels were maintained even 7 days after taurine withdrawal. By contrast, cultures treated with 2 mM of the high-affinity taurine transporter inhibitor guanidinoethanesulfonic acid (GES) showed a sharp decrease in taurine content. When taurine was applied in combination with GES, taurine levels were significantly higher than those observed after GES treatment. Taurine treatment did not affect the relative amount of neurons and oligodendrocytes in the cultures, but promoted the differentiation of O1-positive cells that showed an increase in the length and number of their processes. We conclude that NSC develop specific taurine uptake mechanisms at early stages differentiation. Since taurine was not present in the feeding medium, we suggest that NSC and their progeny have the machinery for taurine synthesis. Present results also indicate that taurine might influence the development of NSC oligodendroglial progeny.

Keywords: neural stem cells, neurospheres, development, taurine, guanidinoethanesulfonic acid, trophic factors

Introduction

Taurine (2-aminoethanesulfonic acid), an end-product of sulphur amino acid catabolism, is a β-amino acid found at high concentrations in several cell types (reviewed in: Huxtable, 1989, 1992; Sturman, 1993). Its zwitterionic nature, at physiological pH, gives high water solubility and low lipophilicity. Thus, the diffusion of taurine across cell membranes does not account for the intracellular levels of this amino acid, which are maintained high from biosynthesis and/or the specific uptake from the extracellular space (Huxtable, 1992). Because taurine does not incorporate into proteins, the greatest proportion of both extracellular and intracellular taurine is in the free form. Several functions have been proposed for this amino acid, such as osmoregulation, membrane stabilization, detoxification, antioxidation, modulation of ion flux, and as a neurotransmitter or neuromodulator and its roles in the control of synaptic transmission have been explored (Thurston et al., 1980; Solís et al., 1988, 1990; Huxtable, 1989, 1992; Galarreta et al., 1996; Schuller-Levis and Park, 2003). Immunohistochemical studies have clarified the cellular localization of taurine in the Central Nervous System (Ottersen et al., 1985; Lake and Verdone-Smith, 1989; Lee et al. 1992; Nagelhus et al., 1993). It has been demonstrated that taurine is essential during retinal development in mammals and potentiates the production of rod photoreceptors by signaling through the glycine receptor GlyRα2 (Renteria et al., 2004; Young and Cepko, 2004). In addition, taurine is the most abundant neurotransmitter in the developing neocortex. During the development of the visual cortex and the cerebellum, it is required for normal ontogeny of neurons. Taurine depletion impairs the migration of cerebellar granule cells in co-cultures of dissociated cerebellum from neonatal mice and neuronal cells (Maar et al., 1995). Sustained taurine deficits during the prenatal and immediate postnatal period result in permanent abnormalities. Taurine-deficient cats have defects that include retinal degeneration, abnormalities of the brain cortex and delayed cerebellar granule cells migration and growth (Strurman et al., 1985; Palackal et al., 1986). All these observations support the notion that taurine is determinant for neural development. However, the moment in which taurine becomes essential for brain development has not been determined, since its possible roles in neural stem/progenitor cells biology is unknown, except for retinal precursor cells.

Neural stem cells are defined as clonogenic cells with self-renewal capacity and the ability to generate all neural lineages. Cells with these characteristics have been isolated from the embryonic and adult Central Nervous System. Under specific conditions, these cells proliferate in cultures as cell clusters called "neurospheres" and differentiate into neurons, glia, and non-neural cell types (reviewed in: Gage, 2000; Kennea and Mehmet, 2002; Bazan et al., 2004). NSC cultures represent a useful model for neurodevelopment studies. Different growth factors, cytokines, extracellular matrix proteins, and neurotransmitters have been implicated in the epigenetic regulation of proliferation and differentiation processes of these cells (Burrows et al., 1997; Arsenijevic and Weiss, 1998; Edlund and Jessell, 1999). Several studies have determined in vitro conditions for promoting the differentiation of NSC into specific cellular phenotypes (Daadi and Weiss, 1999; Reimers et al., 2001; Lopez-Toledano et al., 2004). Here we explore the possibility that taurine could influence the fate determination of neural progenitors in vitro.

Materials and Methods

Differentiation of EGF-expanded neural stem cells

Striatal primordia from E15 Sprage-Dawley rat embryos were dissected and mechanically dissociated. Cell suspensions were grown in a defined medium (DF12) composed of Dulbecco's modified Eagle's medium and Ham's F-12 (1:1), 2 mM L-glutamine, 1 mM sodium piruvate (all from Gibco BRL, Life Technologies Inc, Grand Island, New York), 0.6% glucose, 25 µg/ml insulin, 20 nM progesterone, 60 µM putrescine, and 30 nM sodium selenite (all from Sigma Chemical Co, St Louis, MO), 100 µg/ml human transferrin and 20 ng/ml human recombinant epidermal growth factor (EGF) (both from Boehringer Mannheim GmbH, Germany). The cells grew as floating neurospheres, and were passaged by mechanical dissociation every 2-3 days.

After a minimum of four passages, EGF-expanded NSC (EGF-NSC) were plated at a density of 20,000 to 30,000 cells/cm^2 on 15 µg/ml poly-l-ornithine (Sigma Chemical Co) coated glass coverslips (Ø 12 mm) or plastic dishes (Ø 35 mm). Cultures were maintained in DF12 and 20 ng/ml EGF for 3 days and then switched to DF12 without EGF for longer culture periods (untreated group). At 2 hours post-plating, parallel cultures were treated with 2 mM taurine (TAU), or 2 mM GES (Toronto Research Chemicals Inc., Ontario, Canada), or both (TAU+GES). Immunocytochemical and biochemical analysis were performed at 1, 3, 4 and 10 days post plating (dpp).

Indirect immunocytochemistry

Rabbit polyclonal antibodies and mouse monoclonal antibodies directed against neural antigens, taurine and taurine transporter (TauT) were used as primary antibodies for indirect immunocytochemistry. Polyclonal antibodies against taurine and TauT were purchased from Chemicon International (Temecula, CA) and GFAP from Dakopatts a/s, (Glostrup,

Denmark). Monoclonal antibodies against β-tubulin III were obtained from Sigma Chemical Co. (St. Louis, MO), and anti-nestin (clone Rat 401) and anti-A2B5, O4 and O1 from Developmental Studies Hybridoma Bank (University of Iowa). Secondary antibodies raised in goat against rabbit and in sheep against mouse immunoglobulins, conjugated to lisamine rhodamine (1:100) and fluorescein isothiocyanate (1:100), were purchased from Jackson Immunoresearch Laboratories Inc, (West Grove, PA), and Boehringer Mannheim GmbH, respectively.

For immunocytochemical studies cells were fixed with 4% paraformaldehyde for 10 min and immunostained for A2B5 (1:10), O4 (1:10), O1 (1:10), GFAP (1:500) and β-tubulin III (1:200). For taurine immunostaining, cells were fixed with 2% paraformaldehyde and 0.5% glutaraldehyde. Coverslips were mounted in a medium containing p-phenylenediamine and bisBenzimide (Hoechst 33342, Sigma Chemical Co).

Taurine content determination

Cells on plastic dishes were washed three times in 2 ml of PBS and scraped at 4 °C in 250 μl of 0.2 N perchloric acid - 0.2 mM EDTA - 0.5 mM sodium meta-bisulphite (Na2S2O5). Cell suspensions were sonicated three times for 15 sec and centrifuged at 7200 g x 5 min. The supernatants were frozen at -80 °C until they were analyzed. The pellets were used for protein evaluation. The samples were analyzed for taurine content using the reverse-phase high performance liquid chromatography (HPLC) procedure with O-phthaldialdehide (OPA) precolumn derivatization and fluorimetric detection. This method coincides essentially with that described by Jones and Stein (1981) except that 3-mercaptopropionic acid was used instead of 2-mercaptoethanol in the derivatization reaction. This change improved the sensitivity of the analysis as much as two-fold (Herranz et al., 1985).

Data analysis and cell counting

Results are expressed as the mean ± SEM from 3 independent experiments done in triplicates or quadruplicates. Where indicated, data represent the mean ± SEM of several coverslips. In each coverslip stereological sampling of 25 visual fields (magnification of 200 or 400x) was performed under fluorescence microscopy. The number of cells was corrected for coverslip area. Statistical analyses were performed using Student's t test, or one way ANOVA followed by Bonferoni multiple comparison test and the difference was considered significant when $p \leq 0.05$.

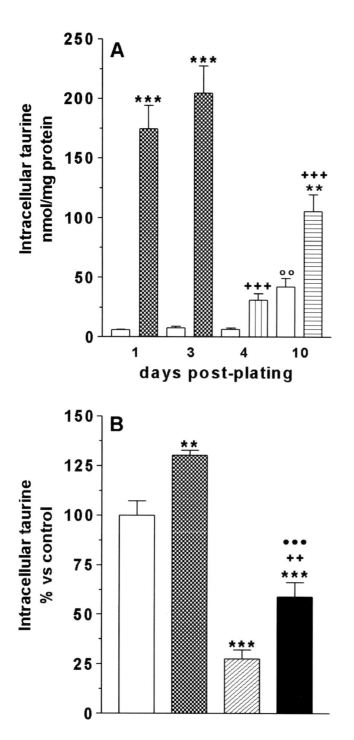

Figure 1.- Taurine levels during the differentiation in vitro of neural stem cells. EGF-expanded neurospheres were plated on plastic dishes in DF12 and 20 ng/ml EGF. In A, 2 hours post-plating neurospheres were treated with vehicle (control) or 2 mM taurine (TAU). Three days later, the medium was switched to DF12 without EGF and cultures were maintained in the absence of any treatment for 1 or 7 additional days. The intracellular content of taurine was measured by HPLC at 1, 3, 4 or 10 days post-plating (dpp). Note the increase in intracellular taurine observed in control cultures at 10 dpp (A, white bars). The intracellular content of the amino acid was significantly increased in those cultures treated for 1 to 3 days with taurine (A, dot bars). Moreover, the intracellular taurine content remained higher than their respective controls after 1 (A, vertical lines bar) or 7 (A, horizontal lines bar) days of taurine withdrawal. In B, 2 hours post-plating neuro-spheres were treated with vehicle (control) (white bar), or 2 mM taurine (TAU) (dot bar), or 2 mM guanidinoethyl sulphonate (GES) (lined bar), or both (TAU+GES) (black bar) and the intracellular taurine content was measured 3 days later by HPLC. Note the decrease in the intracellular content of taurine observed in GES treated cultures (B, lined bar) and the inhibition in taurine uptake observed after 3 days of TAU+GES treatment (B, black bar). Results represent the mean ± ESM of 8 to 12 plates from 3 independent experiments. ** $p \leq 0.01$, *** $p \leq 0.001$ vs. their respective controls. OO $p \leq 0.01$ vs. control at 1 dpp. ++ $p \leq 0.01$, +++ $p \leq 0.001$ vs. 3 dpp TAU treated cultures. ●●● $p \leq 0.001$ vs. 3 dpp GES treated cultures.

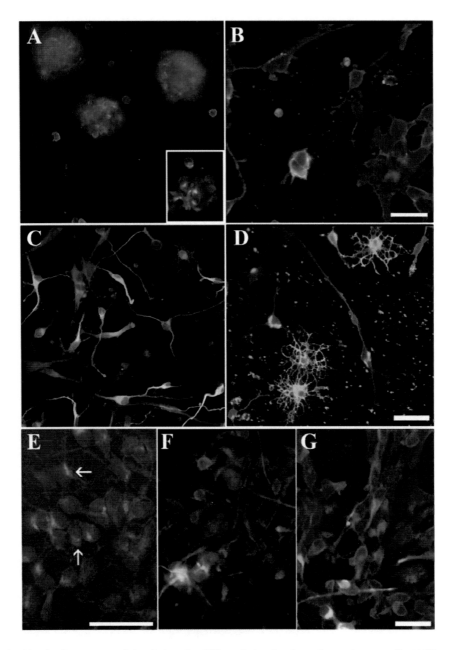

Figure 2.- Taurine immunoreactivity during the differentiation in vitro of neural stem cells. EGF-expanded neurospheres were plated on poly-l-ornithine coated coverslips in DF12 and 20 ng/ml EGF for 3 days. Then, the medium was switched to DF12 without EGF and cultures were maintained for 3 additional days. Double immunostaining for taurine (A-D and F-G, red) and neural antigens was performed at different times post-plating. Taurine-positive cells were observed in recently seeded neurospheres (A, red). Inside the neurospheres some nestin-positive cells (A, green) co-expressed taurine, but taurine and nestin compartments were different (A, insert). At 3 days post-plating (dpp), some A2B5-positive progenitors (B, green) were taurine immuno-positive (B, yellow). At 6 dpp, a subset of β tubulin III-positive (C, green) and O1-positive (D, green) cells co-expressed taurine (C and D, yellow). At 1dpp, EGF-expanded neural stem cells showed taurine transporter immunoreactivity (E, arrows). In F and G, nestin (green) and taurine (red) immunolabeling was analyzed in cultures treated with vehicle (F) or 2 mM taurine (G) for 24 hours. Note the

increase in taurine immunoreactivity promoted by the treatment with the amino acid (G, red). Scale bars, 30 μm.

Results

EGF- expanded neural stem cells synthesize taurine during their differentiation in vitro

EGF-expanded neurospheres were seeded onto adherent substrate and treated with EGF during the first 3 days in culture, in order to enhance the expansion of precursor cells. After this period the mitogen was withdrawn, and cells grew in defined medium. Between 2 hours and 3 dpp cultures comprised mainly nestin-positive undifferentiated precursors (Lobo et al., 2003). As cells are maintained in culture, there is a gradual loss of nestin expression and an increase in the relative content of neurons, oligodendrocytes and astrocytes, as described previously (Bazan et al. 1998; Reimers et al. 2001).

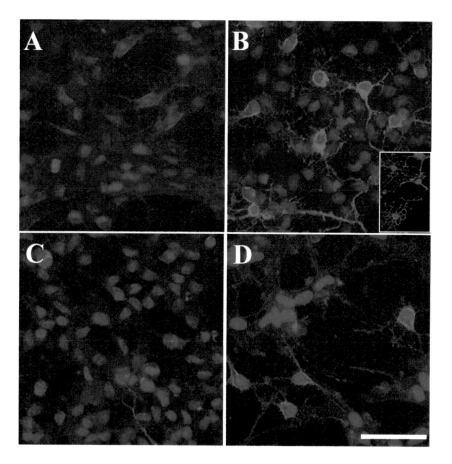

Figure 3.- Neural stem cells express functional taurine transporter in vitro. EGF-expanded neurospheres were plated on poly-l-ornithine coated coverslips in DF12 and 20 ng/ml EGF. At 2 hours post-plating, cultures were treated with vehicle (A), or 2 mM taurine (TAU) (B), or 2 mM guanidinoethyl sulphonate (GES) (C), or both (TAU+GES) (D). Three days later, cultures were fixed and taurine immunoreactivy was analyzed. Taurine imunolabeling was increased in those cultures treated with the amino acid (B, red). Note the increase

in taurine immunoreactivity in the cell processes (B, insert). By contrast, the treatment with GES decreased the number of taurine-positive cells (C, red) as compared with vehicle (A) or TAU treated cultures (B). When taurine was applied in the presence of GES (D, red), taurine immunopositivity was lower than in TAU treated cultures. In blue, cell nuclei labeled with Hoechst. Scale bar, 50 μm.

The intracellular content of taurine was analyzed by HPLC at different times post-plating. At 1 dpp, taurine was detectable at a basal value of 7 nmol/mg protein. This basal value was maintained up to day 4 post-plating, but as cells were further maintained in culture, the intracellular taurine content increased to reach an average value of 40 nmol/mg protein at 10 dpp (Fig. 1A). When the extracellular content of taurine was analyzed, levels from 2 to 5 nmol/plate were detected between 1 to 10 dpp (data not shown). To determine the cell source for taurine in the cultures double-immunostaning studies were performed using specific antibodies directed against neural antigens and taurine. In recently seeded neurospheres (2 hours post-plating), some nestin-positive/taurine-positive cells were observed (Fig. 2A). Between 1 and 3 dpp taurine was detected in nestin-positive and A2B5-positive progenitors (Fig. 2B, F). After 5 dpp, taurine was observed in neurons (Fig. 2C) and oligodendrocytes (Fig. 2D). However, GFAP-positive cells present in the cultures were immunonegative for taurine at any time analyzed (Fig. 4B).

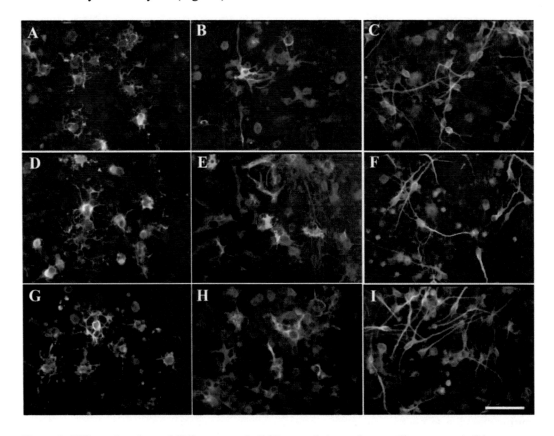

Figure 4.- Effects of taurine and GES treatment in EGF-expanded neural stem cells progeny. At 2 hours post-plating, cultures were treated with vehicle (A, B, C), or 2 mM taurine (D, E, F), or 2 mM guanidinoethyl sulphonate (GES) (G, H, I). Three days later, the medium was switched to DF12 without EGF and cultures were maintained in the absence of any treatment for 7 additional days and double immunostaining analysis for taurine (A-I, red) and O1 (A, D, G, green), GFAP (B, E, H, green) and β tubulin III (C, F, I, green) was performed. Under all experimental conditions, taurine immunoreactivity was observed in O1-positive (A, D,

G, yellow) and β tubulin III-positive cells (C, F, I, yellow) while GFAP-positive cells did not co labeled with taurine (B, E, H). Note that after 7 days of taurine withdrawal oligodendrocytes show a more mature aspect with an increase in their size, and in the length and number of their cellular processes (D). Scale bar, 50 μm.

EGF-expanded neural stem cells express functional taurine transporter during their differentiation in vitro

During the expansive phase (2 hours to 3 dpp), cultures of EGF-NSC showed TauT immunoreactivity (Fig. 2E). To determine whether the addition of exogenous taurine in the culture medium can change its intracellular content, 2 mM taurine was added for 3 days and the cultures were analyzed after 1 and 3 days of treatment, and 1 or 7 days after taurine withdrawal. Taurine immunoreactivity was increased in the cultures after 1or 3 days of treatment with the amino acid (Fig. 2G and Fig. 3B). These results were confirmed when the intracellular taurine content was measured by HPLC (Fig. 1A). One or 7 days after taurine withdrawal, the number of taurine-positive cells in the cultures remained 1.3 to 1.6 fold above controls. At these later experimental times, the intracellular taurine content was lower than during the treatment period (0-3 days), but remained higher than their respective controls (Fig. 1A) confirming the immunocytochemical data. To asses if a mature active taurine transport mechanism is present in these cells, some cultures were treated for the first 3 days with the inhibitor of taurine transporter GES (2 mM) in the absence or presence of 2 mM taurine. The intracellular taurine content was reduced in the cultures after 3 days of GES treatment (Fig. 1B). Taurine-positive cells were also reduced after 3 days of treatment with the inhibitor (Fig. 3C). When taurine was added to EGF-NSC cultures in combination with GES, taurine content was higher than with GES alone, but lower than in control or taurine treated cells (Fig. 1B). Similarly, taurine immunoreactivity was increased in TAU+GES treated cultures as compared with those cultures treated with GES for 3 days (Fig. 3C, D).

Role of taurine in the maturation of oligodendrocytes derived from EGF-neural stem cells

To determine if changes in the intracellular levels of taurine may affect the in vitro differentiation of EGF-NSC, cultures were treated with taurine or GES for 3 days. Double-immunostaning studies were performed 7 days later using specific antibodies directed against neural antigens and taurine. Under all experimental conditions, taurine immunoreactivity was observed in O1-positive (Fig. 4A, D, G) and β tubulin III-positive cells (Fig. 4C, F, I), while no GFAP-positive cells co-labeled with taurine in the cultures (Fig. 4B, E, H). Although no changes in the relative amount of β tubulin III-positive and O1-positive cells were observed (data not shown), the morphology of oligodendrocytes changed in those cultures treated with taurine showing a more mature aspect, with an increase in their size and in the length and number of their cellular processes (Fig. 4D). Interestingly, our immunocytochemical studies performed at 3 dpp showed intense taurine immunoreactivity in cells with the morphology of oligodendrocytes after taurine treatment (Fig. 3B, insert), and this effect was partially prevented by the concomitant treatment with GES (Fig. 3D).

Discussion

Taurine is one of the most abundant amino acid in the brain of mammals, where it is thought to play important roles during development (reviewed in: Sturman, 1993). However, poorly is known about the source of endogenous derived taurine and its transport during the development of neural progenitors. Here we show that taurine can be detected in neural progenitor cells and that active transport mechanisms and biosynthesis of taurine must exist in these cells in vitro. We also show that taurine promotes the maturation of the oligodendrocytes derived from EGF-NSC.

Previously, we reported that recently seeded neurospheres contain detectable levels of taurine (Bazán et al., 1996). Present results show that EGF-NSC maintain relatively high levels of the amino acid during their in vitro differentiation. These result are in agreement with other studies that suggest that taurine is necessary for growth and migration of neural precursors (Maar et al., 1995; Benitez-Diaz e al., 2003). In fact, high levels of taurine were detected in the mouse cerebral cortex during the proliferative stage of neurogenesis, consistent with a possible role as a trophic factor of this amino acid during cortical development. Besides, a protective role for taurine against postnatal excitatory neurotoxicity has been postulated (Benitez-Diaz et al., 2003). Interestingly, the highest levels of intracellular taurine were observed at 10 dpp, a time point when high levels of glutamate are detected in the cultures (Bazan et al., 1996, 1998), as well as the maximal number of neurons and glial cells (Reimers et al., 2001).

In the adult brain, both a glial and a neuronal origin for taurine has been postulated (Dominy et al., 2004). In EGF-NSC, taurine was immunodetected in nestin-positive and A2B5-positive progenitor cells. Because taurine was absent in the feeding medium, the presence of its biosynthetic machinery in neural precursors can be concluded. In our cultures, taurine immunoreactivity was also detected in β tubulin III-positive and O1-positive cells, indicating that neurons and oligodendrocytes derived from these cells are able to synthesize the amino acid. Co- localization of taurine and cysteine sulfinate decarboxylase (CSD), the enzyme that mediates the synthesis of hypotaurine from cysteine, has been described in Purkinje cerebellar neurons (Magnusson et al., 1988). Moreover, in the cerebellum CDS-positive cells were found in the white matter that were typically arranged in rows like oligodendrocytes (Almarghini et al., 1991). Other studies suggest that astrocytes are capable of taurine synthesis (Tappaz et al., 1994; Reymond et al., 1996; Brand et al., 1998). Astrocytes derived from EGF-NSC did not co-labeled with taurine at any time analyzed. The lack of taurine detection could be explained if astrocytes derived from EGF-NSC are only a source for hypotaurine, or if taurine levels in these cells are so low that could not be detected by immunocytochemistry. In addition, it is possible that only mature astrocytes will develop the machinery needed to synthesize hypotaurine and taurine. The use of antibodies to CSD, when commercially available, will be of great value to clarify these observations.

The intracellular taurine concentration is controlled by taurine biosynthetic enzymes and taurine transporters (reviewed in: Lambert, 2004; Tapaz, 2004). Intracellular accumulation of taurine was observed when the amino acid was added to recently seeded EGF-expanded neurospheres indicating that taurine transport mechanisms are present in these cells. High-affinity taurine transports have been described in different brain areas (Smith et al., 1992; Pow et al., 2002). In EGF-NSC, TauT immunoreactivity was observed at early stages of their differentiation in vitro, and the intracellular taurine content was significantly decreased after the chronic administration of the competitive inhibitor of high-affinity taurine transporter GES (Huxtable et al., 1979; Huxtable and Lippincott, 1981). Moreover, taurine uptake was partially inhibited by the inhibitor. Altogether these results indicate that EGF-NSC must express a high-affinity taurine transporter. Other studies reported that 100 μM GES is sufficient for a 70% inhibition of the TauT activity in cultures of Bergmann glial cells (Barakat et al., 2002) and 2mM GES completely inhibit the taurine transport in astrocytes and neurons from the mouse cerebellum (Moran and Pasantes-Morales, 1991). We used 2 mM GES, so a nearly complete inhibition of TauT was expected. However, as we already mentioned, taurine uptake was significantly reduced but not completely abolished by GES. These results suggest that additional taurine transport mechanisms might be present in the cultures. Taurine can activate equally TauT and GABA transporter (GABAT) but high concentrations (1.3 to 2.9 mM) are required for 50% of taurine uptake via GABAT (Sivakami et al., 1992; Liu et al., 1993; Borden., 1996; Sergeeva et al., 2003). Since we use taurine at a concentration of 2 mM, a GABAT mediated transport can not be excluded. Taurine can be also transported by low-affinity transport systems in the brain and retina (Saransaari and Oja, 1992, Sanchez-Olea et al., 1993, Martin del Rio and Solis, 1998, Militante and Lombardini, 1999). It is plausible that a low-affinity transport system might serve to accumulate taurine in EGF-NSC. In the future, the presence and identity of this low-affinity transport system will be studied.

Taurine uptake has been identified in mature neurons and glial cells including oligodendrocytes (Reynolds and Herschkowithz 1986; Walz and Allen, 1987; Della Corte et al., 1990; Kritzer et al., 1992; Pow et al., 2002; Walz, 2002). According to our immunocytochemical results, nestin-positive neural precursors also have the ability to accumulate taurine when the amino acid was added to the culture medium. On the other hand, high levels of the amino acid were observed in the neuronal and oligodendroglial progeny after taurine treatment. Because no mature neurons and oligodendrocytes are present in the cultures at the time point when taurine is applied, we may argue that taurine transport mechanisms must be expressed by their progenitors. It is noteworthy that changes in the intracellular taurine content increase the size of the oligodendrocytes derived from EGF-NSC and the length and number of their cellular processes. Although taurine stimulates neurite outgrowth in neurons (Chen et al., 1998; Lima, 1999), to our knowledge this is the first study showing a trophic effect of taurine in oligodendrocytes. The fact that these effects were partially prevented by the concomitant treatment of taurine with GES (Fig. 3D) suggest that the high-affinity taurine transporter mediates, at least in part, this action of the amino acid. On the other hand, taurine could stimulate the differentiation of oligodendrocytes by acting on Glycine receptors (GlyRs). Taurine is a ligand of GABA receptors (GABAR) and GlyRs (Haas and Hosli, 1973; Hussy et al., 1997; Sergeeva and Haas, 2001; Barakat et al., 2002), and GlyRs have been proposed as mediators for the functions of taurine during brain development (Flint et al., 1998). GlyRs have been described in cultured oligodendrocyte progenitors (Belachew et al., 1998) and high levels of Glycine were detected in EGF-NSC during their differentiation in vitro (Bazan et al., 1996, 1998). Moreover, similarly than taurine GES is able to interact with GlyRs and $GABA_A R$ in cultures of neurons (Sergeeva et al., 2002; Herranz et al., 1990).

We conclude that NSC develop specific taurine uptake mechanisms at early stages of their differentiation in vitro. Moreover, NSC and their neuronal and oligodendroglial progeny have the machinery needed for taurine synthesis. The present study also indicates that taurine probably acts as a trophic factor on oligodendrocytes derived from NSC. While these findings suggest a role of taurine on the development of NSC, further experiments are needed to better understand the functions of this factor.

Acknowledgments

This work was supported by Fondo de Investigaciones Sanitarias (FIS 97/0269 and FIS 02/0853) and Raquel Alonso by Fundación MAPFRE Medicina. We are grateful to Dr. Rafael Martín del Río (Servicio de Neurolobiología-Invetigación, Hospital Ramón y Cajal, Madrid, Spain) for comments and critical reading of this manuscript.

References

Almarghini K, Remy A, Tappaz M. *Immunocytochemistry of the taurine biosynthesis enzyme, cysteine sulfinate decarboxylase, in the cerebellum: evidence for a glial localization.*

Arsenijevic Y, Weiss S. Insulin-like growth factor-I is a differentiation factor for postmitotic CNS stem cell-derived neuronal precursors: distinct actions from those of brain-derived neurotrophic factor. *J Neurosci.* 1998, 18:2118-2128.

Barakat L, Wang D, Bordey A. Carrier-mediated uptake and release of taurine from Bergmann glia in rat cerebellar slices. *J Physiol.* 2002, 541:753-67.

Bazan E, Alonso FJ, Redondo C et al. In vitro and in vivo characterization of neural stem cells. *Histol Histopathol.* 2004, 19:1261-75.

Bazan E, Lopez-Toledano MA, Mena MA, Martín del Rio R, Paino CL and Herranz A S. *Endogenous Amino Acid Profile During In Vitro Differentiation of Neural Stem Cells.* In Fiskum G, ed. Neurodegenerative Diseases. New York, Plenum Press, 1996, 225-234.

Bazan E, Lopez-Toledano MA, Redondo C, Alcazar A, Paino CL, Herranz AS. *Characterization of rat neural stem cells from embryonic striatum and mesencephalon during in vitro differentiation.* In Castellano B, González B, Nieto-Sampedro M, eds. Understanding Glial Cells. Dordrecht, Kluwer Academic Publishers, 1998, 133-147.

Belachew S, Rogister B, Rigo JM, Malgrange B, Mazy-Servais C, Xhauflaire G, Coucke P, Moonen G. Cultured oligodendrocyte progenitors derived from cerebral cortex express a glycine receptor which is pharmacologically distinct from the neuronal isoform. *Eur J Neurosci.* 1998; 10:3556-64.

Benitez-Diaz P, Miranda-Contreras L, Mendoza-Briceno RV, Pena-Contreras Z, Palacios-Pru E. Prenatal and postnatal contents of amino acid neurotransmitters in mouse parietal cortex. *Dev Neurosci.* 2003, 25:366-374.

Borden LA. GABA transporter heterogeneity: pharmacology and cellular localization. *Neurochem Int.* 1996, 29:335-356.

Brand A, Leibfritz D, Hamprecht B, Dringen R. Metabolism of cysteine in astroglial cells: synthesis of hypotaurine and taurine. *J Neurochem.* 1998, 71:827-32.

Burrows RC, Wancio D, Levitt P, Lillien L. Response diversity and the timing of progenitor cell maturation are regulated by developmental changes in EGFR expression in the cortex. *Neuron* 1997, 19:251-267.

Chen XC, Pan ZL, Liu DS, Han X. Effect of taurine on human fetal neuron cells: proliferation and differentiation. *Adv Exp Med Biol.* 1998; 442:397-403.

Daadi MM, Weiss S. Generation of tyrosine hydroxylase-producing neurons from precursors of the embryonic and adult forebrain. *J Neurosci.* 1999, 19:4484-4497.

Della Corte L, Bolam JP, Clarke DJ, Parry DM, Smith AD. Sites of [3H]taurine Uptake in the Rat Substantia Nigra in Relation to the Release of Taurine from the Striatonigral Pathway. *Eur J Neurosci.* 1990, 2:50-61.

Dominy J, Eller S, Dawson R Jr. Building biosynthetic schools: reviewing compartmentation of CNS taurine synthesis. *Neurochem Res.* 2004, 29:97-103.

Edlund T, Jessell TM. Progression from extrinsic to intrinsic signaling in cell fate specification: a view from the nervous system. *Cell* 1999, 96:211-224.

Flint AC, Liu X, Kriegstein AR. Nonsynaptic glycine receptor activation during early neocortical development. *Neuron* 1998, 20: 43-53.

Gage FH. Mammalian neural stem cells. *Science* 2000; 287:1433-8.

Galarreta M, Bustamante J, Martin del Rio R, Solis JM. Taurine induces a long-lasting increase of synaptic efficacy and axon excitability in the hippocampus. *J Neurosci.* 1996, 16: 92-102.

Haas HL, Hosli L. The depression of brain stem neurones by taurine and its interaction with strychnine and bicuculline. *Brain Res.* 1973, 52:399-402.

Herranz , A.S., Cristín, J. L., Lerma, J. and Martín del Rio, R.. Incremento de sensibilidad en los análisis por CLAE de los OPA-amioácidos usando como reactivo de derivación el ácido 3-mercapto-propiónico. Resúmenes de la Reunión Científica anual del grupo de Cromatografía y Tecnicas afines, *RSEQ.* 1985, 58-59.

Herranz AS, Solis JM, Herreras O, Menendez N, Ambrosio E, Orensanz LM, Martin del Rio R. The epileptogenic action of the taurine analogue guanidinoethane sulfonate may be caused by a blockade of GABA receptors. *J Neurosci Res.* 1990, 26:98-104.

Hussy N, Deleuze C, Pantaloni A, Desarmenien MG, Moos F. Agonist action of taurine on glycine receptors in rat supraoptic magnocellular neurones: possible role in osmoregulation. *J Physiol.* 1997, 502:609-621.

Huxtable RJ. Taurine in the central nervous system and the mammalian actions of taurine. *Prog Neurobiol.* 1989, 32:471-533.

Huxtable RJ. Physiological actions of taurine. *Physiol Rev.* 1992, 72:101-163.

Huxtable RJ, Laird HE 2nd, Lippincott SE. The transport of taurine in the heart and the rapid depletion of tissue taurine content by guanidinoethyl sulfonate. *J Pharmacol Exp Ther.* 1979; 211:465-71.

Huxtable RJ, Lippincott SE. Sources and turnover rates of taurine in newborn, weanling, and mature rats. *Adv Exp Med Biol.* 1981;139:23-45.

Jones B N, Stein S. Amino acid analysis and enzymatic sequence determination of peptides by an improved O-phthaldialdehyde precolumn lavelling procedure. *J. Liquid Chromatogr.* 1981, 4: 565-586.

Kennea NL, Mehmet H. Neural stem cells. *J Pathol.* 2002 Jul;197(4):536-50.

Kritzer MF, Cowey A, Ottersen OP, Streit P, Somogyi P. Immunoreactivity for Taurine Characterizes Subsets of Glia, GABAergic and non-GABAergic Neurons in the Neo- and

Archicortex of the Rat, Cat and Rhesus Monkey: Comparison with Immunoreactivity for Homocysteic Acid. *Eur J Neurosci.* 1992; 4:251-270.

Lake N, Verdone-Smith C. Immunocytochemical localization of taurine in the mammalian retina. *Curr Eye Res.* 1989, 8:163-173.

Lambert IH. Regulation of the cellular content of the organic osmolyte taurine in mammalian cells. *Neurochem Res.* 2004; 29:27-63.

Lee IS, Renno WM, Beitz AJ. A quantitative light and electron microscopic analysis of taurine-like immunoreactivity in the dorsal horn of the rat spinal cord. *J Comp Neurol.* 1992, 321:65-82.

Lima L. Taurine and its trophic effects in the retina. *Neurochem Res.* 1999; 24:1333-8.

Liu QR, Lopez-Corcuera B, Mandiyan S, Nelson H, Nelson N. Molecular characterization of four pharmacologically distinct gamma-aminobutyric acid transporters in mouse brain. *J Biol Chem.* 1993, 268:2106-2112.

Lobo MV, Alonso FJ, Redondo C, Lopez-Toledano MA, Caso E, Herranz AS, Paino CL, Reimers D, Bazan E. Cellular characterization of epidermal growth factor-expanded free-floating neurospheres. *J Histochem Cytochem.* 2003, 51: 89-103.

Lopez-Toledano MA, Redondo C, Lobo MV, Reimers D, Herranz AS, Paino CL, Bazan E.Tyrosine hydroxylase induction by basic fibroblast growth factor and cyclic AMP analogs in striatal neural stem cells: role of ERK1/ERK2 mitogen-activated protein kinase and protein kinase C. *J Histochem Cytochem.* 2004, 52:1177-1189.

Maar T, Moran J, Schousboe A, Pasantes-Morales H. Taurine deficiency in dissociated mouse cerebellar cultures affects neuronal migration. *Int J Dev Neurosci.* 1995, 13:491-502

Magnusson KR, Madl JE, Clements JR, Wu JY, Larson AA, Beitz AJ. Colocalization of taurine- and cysteine sulfinic acid decarboxylase-like immunoreactivity in the cerebellum of the rat with monoclonal antibodies against taurine. *J Neurosci.* 1988, 8:4551-4564.

Martin del Rio R, Solis JM. The anion-exchanger AE1 is a diffusion pathway for taurine transport in rat erythrocytes. *Adv Exp Med Biol.* 1998; 442:255-60.

Militante JD, Lombardini JB. Taurine uptake activity in the rat retina: protein kinase C-independent inhibition by chelerythrine. *Brain Res.* 1999; 818:368-74.

Moran J, Pasantes-Morales H. Taurine-deficient cultured cerebellar astrocytes and granule neurons obtained by treatment with guanidinoethane sulfonate. *J Neurosci Res.* 1991, 29:533-537.

Nagelhus EA, Lehmann A, Ottersen OP.Neuronal-glial exchange of taurine during hypo-osmotic stress: a combined immunocytochemical and biochemical analysis in rat cerebellar cortex. *Neuroscience* 1993, 54:615-631.

Ottersen OP, Madsen S, Meldrum BS, Storm-Mathisen J. Taurine in the hippocampal formation of the Senegalese baboon, Papio papio: an immunocytochemical study with an antiserum against conjugated taurine. *Exp Brain Res.* 1985, 59:457-462.

Palackal T, Moretz R, Wisniewski H, Sturman J. Abnormal visual cortex development in the kitten associated with maternal dietary taurine deprivation. *J Neurosci Res.* 1986, 15:223-239.

Pow DV, Sullivan R, Reye P, Hermanussen S. Localization of taurine transporters, taurine, and (3)H taurine accumulation in the rat retina, pituitary, and brain. *Glia.* 2002, 37:153-168.

Reimers D, Lopez-Toledano MA, Mason I, Cuevas P, Redondo C, Herranz AS, Lobo MV, Bazan E. Developmental expression of fibroblast growth factor (FGF) receptors in neural stem cell progeny. Modulation of neuronal and glial lineages by basic FGF treatment. *Neurol Res.* 2001, 23:612-621.

Renteria RC, Johnson J, Copenhagen DR. Need rods? Get glycine receptors and taurine. *Neuron* 2004, 41:839-41.

Reymond I; Almarghini K, Tappaz M. Immunocytochemical localization of cysteine sulfinate decarboxylase in astrocytes in the cerebellum and hippocampus: a quantitative double immunofluorescence study with glial fibrillary acidic protein and S-100 protein. *Neuroscience* 1996, 75:619-33.

Reynolds R, Herschkowitz N. Selective uptake of neuroactive amino acids by both oligodendrocytes and astrocytes in primary dissociated culture: a possible role for oligodendrocytes in neurotransmitter metabolism. *Brain Res.* 1986, 371:253-66.

Sanchez-Olea R, Pena C, Moran J, Pasantes-Morales H. Inhibition of volume regulation and efflux of osmoregulatory amino acids by blockers of Cl- transport in cultured astrocytes. *Neurosci Lett.* 1993, 156:141-144.

Saransaari P, Oja SS. Taurine transport in the mouse cerebral cortex during development and ageing. *Adv Exp Med Biol.* 1992;315:215-20.

Schuller-Levis GB, Park E. Taurine: new implications for an old amino acid. *FEMS Microbiol Lett.* 2003;226:195-202.

Sergeeva OA, Chepkova AN, Doreulee N, Eriksson KS, Poelchen W, Monnighoff I, Heller-Stilb B, Warskulat U, Haussinger D, Haas HL. Taurine-induced long-lasting enhancement of synaptic transmission in mice: role of transporters. *J Physiol.* 2003, 550:911-919.

Sergeeva OA, Chepkova AN, Haas HL.Guanidinoethyl sulphonate is a glycine receptor antagonist in striatum. *Br J Pharmacol.* 2002, 137:855-60.

Sergeeva OA, Haas HL. Expression and function of glycine receptors in striatal cholinergic interneurons from rat and mouse. *Neuroscience* 2001, 104:1043-1055.

Sivakami S, Ganapathy V, Leibach FH, Miyamoto Y. The gamma-aminobutyric acid transporter and its interaction with taurine in the apical membrane of the bovine retinal pigment epithelium. *Biochem J.* 1992, 283:391-397.

Smith KE, Borden LA, Wang CH, Hartig PR, Branchek TA, Weinshank RL. Cloning and expression of a high affinity taurine transporter from rat brain. *Mol Pharmacol.* 1992, 42:563-569.

Solis JM, Herranz AS, Herreras O, Lerma J, Martin del Rio R. Does taurine act as an osmoregulatory substance in the rat brain? *Neurosci Lett.* 1988, 91:53-58.

Solis JM, Herranz AS, Herreras O, Menendez N, del Rio RM. Weak organic acids induce taurine release through an osmotic-sensitive process in in vivo rat hippocampus. *J Neurosci Res.* 1990, 26:159-167.

Sturman J A. Taurine in development. *Physiol Rev.* 1993, 73:119-47.

Sturman JA, Moretz RC, French JH, Wisniewski HM. Taurine deficiency in the developing cat: persistence of the cerebellar external granule cell layer. *J Neurosci Res.* 1985; 13:405-416.

Tappaz M, Almarghini K, Do K. Cysteine sulfinate decarboxylase in brain: identification, characterization and immunocytochemical location in astrocytes. *Adv Exp Med Biol.* 1994, 359:257-268.

Tappaz ML. Taurine biosynthetic enzymes and taurine transporter: molecular identification and regulations. *Neurochem Res.* 2004;29:83-96.

Thurston JH, Hauhart RE, Dirgo JA. Taurine: a role in osmotic regulation of mammalian brain and possible clinical significance. *Life Sci.* 1980, 26:1561-1568.

Young, TL, Cepko CL. A role for ligand-gated ion channels in rod photoreceptor development. *Neuron* 2004, 41:867-879.

Walz W. Chloride/anion channels in glial cell membranes. Glia. 2002; 40:1-10.

Walz W, Allen AF. Evaluation of the osmoregulatory function of taurine in brain cells. *Exp Brain Res.* 1987; 68:290-8.

In: Neural Stem Cell Research
Editor: Eric V. Grier, pp. 115-153

ISBN: 1-59454-846-3
© 2006 Nova Science Publishers, Inc.

Chapter 6

RETROVIRUS VECTOR SILENCING IN STEM CELLS

*Shuyuan Yao and James Ellis**

Developmental Biology Program
Hospital for Sick Children
555 University Ave. Toronto
Ontario, Canada M5G 1X8
and Department of Molecular & Medical Genetics
University of Toronto

Abstract

Retrovirus vectors suffer severe gene silencing in stem cells that hampers their use in stem cell gene therapy. Transduced retrovirus vector can be completely silenced, or dynamically silenced in a subset of cells resulting in variegation. Expressing retrovirus also can be extinguished during stem cell differentiation. Multiple epigenetic modifications including histone modifications and DNA methylation are functionally involved in establishing and maintaining retrovirus silencing via the formation of silent chromatin. A model is proposed that the balance of epigenetic effects at the integration site and retroviral silencer elements on the vectors determines the decision to be silent, variegated or expressing in stem cells. Silencing resistant retrovirus vectors have been developed by removal of these silencer elements, and silencing in stem cells may ultimately be blocked using appropriate insulator elements.

Gene therapy holds the potential to treat cancer, inherited or acquired monogenic disorders and other diseases. A broad arsenal of gene transfer systems is currently available and is still expanding. Among them, the retrovirus vector system has attracted a lot of interest for high efficiency transfer into a wide range of cell types and stable integration into the host genome. Because of their ability to repopulate an entire system, stem cells are often targets

---

* Corresponding author: James Ellis, Tel: 416-813-7295; Fax: 416-813-8883; E-mail: jellis@sickkids.ca

for therapeutic gene delivery. The use of retrovirus vectors has been particularly valuable for introducing and expressing foreign genes in stem cells, for genetic marking of stem cells to trace their differentiation and for mutating and tagging genes associated with specific phenotypes. However, the use of retrovirus vectors has been significantly hampered by gene silencing of retrovirus vector expression in primitive cell types such as embryonic stem (ES) cells, embryonal carcinoma (EC) cells, hematopoietic stem cells (HSC) and early embryos. Understanding retrovirus vector silencing and its mechanisms will benefit the development of retrovirus based stem cell gene transfer vectors and the design of stem cell based gene therapy strategies.

1. Background and phenomena

1.1. Retrovirus silencing

Retrovirus silencing was documented as early as 1975 in the study of Moloney Murine Leukemia Virus (Mo-MuLV) infection of 4-8 cell stage mouse preimplantation embryos [Jaenisch et al., 1975]. Although one of the animals raised from infected embryos developed leukemia, no virus was detected from the infected embryos by both co-cultivated viral infection plaque forming assay and electron microscopy. Preimplantation mouse embryos are susceptible to virus integration but cannot express viral functions. In contrast, midgestation stage embryos or newborn mice can be successfully infected by Mo-MuLV and produce viral proteins [Jaenisch, 1980]. Non-virus-producing cell lines derived from a mouse embryo carrying a genetically transmitted Mo-MuLV genome can be reactivated by 5-bromodeoxyuridine (BrdU) to express viral p30 protein in almost all the cells and produce infectious virus in some of the cells [Bacheler et al., 1979]. Clearly, there is a block in preimplantation embryos making them non-permissive to Mo-MuLV gene expression and viral production.

Murine embryonic carcinoma (EC) cells share with preimplantation embryos the potential to differentiate into all three germinal layer cells [Illmensee and Mintz, 1976]. EC cells have been used as an *in vitro* model to study retrovirus silencing in preimplantation embryos. Among the many publications describing retrovirus silencing in EC cells [Gautsch, 1980; Peries et al., 1977; Teich et al., 1977], Speers et al convincingly demonstrated it by picking single cell clones from Mo-MuLV infected EC cells [Speers et al., 1980]. While viral protein and viral production were never observed in undifferentiated EC cells, after differentiation and BrdU drug treatment 2 of 4 clones were reactivated to express viral p30 protein and produce virus particles. The reactivation indicates that retrovirus can be infected into EC cells and that the lack of viral production is due to a block in retrovirus expression. Comparison of the same retrovirus infection in EC cells and differentiated cells is a useful model to study retrovirus silencing.

The features of retrovirus silencing can be summarized as being most prevalent in primitive cells, heritable and transcriptional. Both preimplantation embryo cells and EC cells are primitive cells in their early differentiation stages. Other more differentiated cells are permissive for retrovirus expression indicating that retrovirus silencing is primitive cell type specific. Silent retrovirus is kept silenced during culture, during *in vitro* and *in vivo* differentiation, and even during passage from generation to generation. Therefore, the silenced retrovirus state is heritable. The silent provirus genome is intact and functional [Speers et al., 1980; Stewart et al., 1982]. Retrovirus silencing happens after viral integration and before mRNA translation. In fact, Gautsch and Wilson showed that retrovirus expressing EC cells produce 400-700 fold higher virus based nascent RNA than silent EC cells [Gautsch and Wilson, 1983]. Obviously, transcriptional gene silencing plays an important role in retrovirus silencing, although post-transcriptional silencing of retrovirus has been reported in differentiated cells [Gao et al., 2002].

1.2. Retrovirus vector silencing

Retrovirus vectors are derived from isolated retroviruses to transfer and integrate foreign genes into target cells. Retrovirus vectors are created by removing viral genes, leaving only the cis-acting sequences necessary for a single round of replication to avoid vector multiplication and spread to other cells [Buchschacher and Wong-Staal, 2000]. Retrovirus silencing was originally observed with infectious retrovirus. With the development of retrovirus vectors, more and more vectors with easily detectable reporter genes have been used in stem cells gene transfer. The use of retrovirus vectors extends retrovirus silencing studies into other types of primitive cells such as embryonic stem (ES) cells [Cherry et al., 2000; Laker et al., 1998], hematopoietic stem cells (HSC) [Challita and Kohn, 1994; Klug et al., 2000; Lange and Blankenstein, 1997] and hematopoietic progenitor cells [Zentilin et al., 2000]. Retrovirus vector silencing is also found in human SRCs (SCID repopulating cells, a type of HSC), confirming that retroviral silencing occurs in humans and thus will likely pose a significant problem to clinical application of retroviral mediated gene therapy [Guenechea et al., 2001]. The use of retrovirus vectors helped to identify several types of retrovirus vector silencing phenomena. In the literature, retrovirus vector silencing has referred to any phenomena related to non-expression of genes from an integrated retrovirus vector. In the early retrovirus silencing studies, Mo-MuLV was extensively used. Since Mo-MuLV induces severe silencing in EC cells, those studies were focused on silencing established directly after viral infection. Later studies using wildtype or modified retrovirus vectors found the existence of variegated expression and extinction during differentiation or long-term culture.

1.2.1. Retrovirus vector variegation

Retrovirus vectors can be silenced at different levels. The most extreme example is that the retrovirus vector is totally shut down with no transgene expression. Less well known is that it can be variegated in which retrovirus integrated at the same integration site is either silent or expressing (Figure 1). Single cell derived clones picked from MESV based vector transduced murine ES cells showed a varied percentage of positive cells among different clones and varied expression level among cells in the same clone [Laker et al., 1998]. Variegation of the MSCV retrovirus vector in transduced ES cells was also reported by Christopher Klug's laboratory [Swindle et al., 2004]. In their work about 35% (21 out of 55) of the integrated provirus showed variegated expression. An interesting feature of variegated

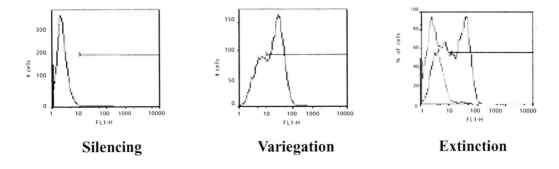

Silencing   **Variegation**   **Extinction**

Figure 1. Retrovirus vector silencing, variegation and extinction in embryonic stem cells. Flow cytometry for eGFP expression shows retrovirus vector silencing, variegation and extinction. While silent retrovirus does not express in any cells, variegated retrovirus expresses in some cells but is silent in others. In extinction, a variegated retrovirus in ES cells (dotted line) is silenced after differentiation (solid line) [Yao, 2004].

retrovirus is instability. Sorted expressing and non-expressing cells from the variegated clones revert to the variegated expression pattern after brief expansion [Swindle et al., 2004]. Clones picked from a variegated clone by limit dilution are also variegated (Yao, S. et al., unpublished data). Unstable variegated clones were also isolated from retrovirus transduced de novo methylase null (dnmt3a-/-3b-/-) ES cells [Yao, 2004]. Therefore, variegation represents a dynamic silencing phenomenon occurring on some of the integrated retroviral proviruses in ES cells. Variegated expression was also observed in retrovirus vector transduced hematopoietic progenitor cell clones [Zentilin et al., 2000].

The expressing and non-expressing cells of the variegated clones contain the same retrovirus vector with the same integration site. Reactivation of the non-expressing cells with 5-AzaC in wildtype variegated ES cells further shows that the retrovirus vector in these cells is intact and functional [Yao, 2004]. Therefore, variegated retrovirus expression is due to epigenetic regulation.

1.2.2. Retrovirus vector extinction after long-term culture

Retrovirus silencing can occur at different time points. Retrovirus expression can be shut down immediately post-integration which results in no transgene expression at any time. In silent preimplantation embryos no virus production was observed from both co-culture plaque forming assay and electron microscopy [Jaenisch et al., 1975]. With EC cells, the nascent RNA produced in silent EC cells is the same as uninfected EC cell control [Niwa et al., 1983]. This kind of silencing is also observed in ES cells [Laker et al., 1998] and long-term HSC cells [Klug et al., 2000]. In contrast, retrovirus that initially express may be silenced in a process known as extinction (Figure 1). Extinction is often observed after long term culture. For example, a GFP retrovirus vector is subject to extinction where both the percentage of cells that are GFP positive and the GFP expression level decrease in transduced murine ES cells after 26 days of passage and culture [Cherry et al., 2000]. Retrovirus vector extinction was also observed in hematopoietic cell lines [McInerney et al., 2000]. Long-term extinction also occurs *in vivo*. Mo-MuLV based retrovirus vector transduced HSC can be assayed as colony forming units-spleen (CFU-S) generated after serial transplantation of infected born marrow cells. While high level gene expression was achieved in all of the primary CFU-S and tissues of the reconstituted marrow transplantation recipients, vector expression is inactive in >90% of the secondary CFU-S and 100% of the third CFU-S [Challita and Kohn, 1994]. Since the primary CFU-S is derived from a committed progenitor cell restricted to the myeloid lineage, this result suggests retrovirus vector in HSC cells is extinguished during serial transplantation. Interestingly, stable transgene expression can be achieved after long-term culture. The factors that control the decision for long-term transgene extinction are not yet clear.

1.2.3. Retrovirus vector extinction after differentiation

In vivo and *in vitro* differentiation of retrovirus vector infected primitive cells can also induce extinction of transgene expression. MESV based retrovirus vector transduced ES cell clones are subject to extinction after *in vitro* differentiation. This was observed with two different reporter genes (LacZ and IL3neoR) and in two different ES cell lines (W9.5 and R1). MESV vector expression was also extinguished after *in vivo* differentiation by making ES cell derived embryos [Laker et al., 1998]. Extinction of retrovirus vectors was also reported after differentiation of HSC. Retrovirus vector expression in transduced long-term HSC was extinguished when differentiated into lymphoid cell populations after transplantation [Klug et al., 2000]. When retrovirus transduced ES cell clones were subjected to 8 days *in vitro* differentiation, extinction occurred primarily on the variegated clones [Yao, 2004], suggesting retrovirus extinction during differentiation may be a consequence of variegation.

1.2.4. Implications of retrovirus vector silencing

Retrovirus vector silencing is a heterogeneous phenomena. The existence of different kinds of silencing on retrovirus vectors implies that a constant monitoring system exists in cells to ensure genomic integrity. The identification of these different retrovirus silencing phenomena are beneficial in terms of evaluating new designs for retrovirus vectors and new gene therapy strategies. Because most of the *ex vivo* transplantation experiments use expressing cells obtained by drug selection or FACS sorting, variegated expressing cells are not excluded. The existence of the unstable variegated expressing cells and their extinction during differentiation may account for some of the unsuccessful gene therapy transplants. Therefore, methods should be developed to distinguish expressing cells and variegated expressing cells before therapeutic transplantation.

1.3. Lentivirus vector silencing

1.3.1. Lentivirus vector

The newest and perhaps most promising vectors developed for the infection of non-dividing quiescent stem cells are Lentiviral vectors. Lentivirus vectors gained popularity since Naldini et al [Naldini et al., 1996] demonstrated in 1996 that human immunodeficiency virus type 1 (HIV-1) based vectors were capable of transducing nondividing cells. Conventional retrovirus vectors are limited by their inability to infect terminally differentiated and nondividing cell types. Lentivirus vectors do not rely on the passive mechanism of nuclear envelope breakdown during the cell cycle to gain entry to the nucleus. Instead they utilize active transport mechanisms and achieve entry through the nucleopore [Chicurel, 2000]. This feature is particularly relevant when infecting slowly dividing stem cells, because a greater transduction efficiency is achieved in comparison to Mo-MuLV based retroviruses [Uchida et al., 1998]. Experiments with Lentiviruses have shown that they are able to efficiently transduce human SRCs [Schilz et al., 1998; Woods et al., 2000], which will be necessary for extending findings in mice to clinical trials.

Like Mo-MuLV, HIV-1 was selected for deriving gene transfer vectors for its well understood viral biology and extensively studied molecular biology. Other Lentiviruses also have been used to develop gene transfer vectors [Quinonez and Sutton, 2002]. Three refinements have been achieved to improve HIV-1 based Lentivirus vector usability and especially safety: Lentivirus vector particle pseudotyping, improvement of the packaging constructs and cell lines [Dull et al., 1998; Kim et al., 1998; Naldini et al., 1996; Naldini and Verma, 2000; Zufferey et al., 1997], and self-inactivating deletions in SIN-Lentivirus vector LTRs [Iwakuma et al., 1999; Miyoshi et al., 1998; Zufferey et al., 1998]. Other cis-acting elements such as the central polypurine tract (cppt) [Sirven et al., 2000; Sirven et al., 2001], Rev response element (RRE) [May et al., 2000] and woodchuck posttranscriptional element (WPRE) [Zufferey et al., 1999] were also included into Lentivirus vectors to improve viral titer or viral expression.

1.3.2. Lentivirus vector silencing

Lentivirus is subject to some gene silencing effects in primitive cells. Lentivirus vector silencing was documented in transduced murine hematopoietic progenitor cells. Primitive hematopoietic progenitor cells were transduced with HIV-1 based Lentivirus vector expressing the green fluorescent protein (GFP) gene and then plated for hematopoietic progenitor cell assays. The primary colonies formed are mosaic for GFP expression. When secondary colonies were cultured from the primary colonies 13% of them are GFP negative while PCR analysis showed the existence of Lentivirus provirus [Mikkola et al., 2000]. While this report showed that Lentivirus vector silencing occurs at least at the progenitor stage, we reported Lentivirus silencing in ES cells by identification of silent single copy vector transduced ES cell clone [Yao, 2004]. Lentivirus was also reported to extinguish during ES cell differentiation into CD34+ hematopoietic progenitor cells [Hamaguchi et al., 2000; Ma et al., 2003].

Some reports suggest there is no gene silencing in Lentivirus vector transduced primitive cells and during their differentiation [Lois et al., 2002; Pfeifer et al., 2002]. In Pfeifer's work, a SIN Lentivirus vector with *cppt* and WPRE was used to harbor either PGK or CAG (contains a modified chicken β-actin promoter and enhancer sequence from cytomegalovirus) promoter driven eGFP or LacZ genes. With multiplicity of infection (moi) of 5, about 50% of the cells are GFP positive with an integrated provirus copy of 1 to 3. An moi of 50 was needed to reach 100% positive cells in both murine and human ES cells. Transduced ES cell colonies stayed GFP positive when differentiated into EBs *in vitro* and into teratomas *in vivo*. Transduced ES cells can be readily used to make chimeras by blastocyst injection, and transgene expression was achieved in most of the organs and transmitted through the germ line. Infected eight-cell stage embryos showed transgene expression after 48 hours and expression continued during embryogenesis and after birth. Lois also reported that Lentivirus vectors escaped developmental silencing during embryogenesis [Lois et al., 2002].

Copy number differences may account for the conflicting observations on Lentivirus vector silencing. Multiple provirus copies can exist in one cell and an expressing provirus can mask silent provirus in the same cell. Single cell clones with a single functionally intact provirus are the ideal systems for Lentivirus silencing studies.

1.4. Retrovirus silencing is epigenetic

Epigenetics by definition is "the study of mitotically and/or meiotically heritable changes in the function of a gene that cannot be explained by changes in its DNA sequences" [Russo, 1996]. Epigenetic regulation plays a key role in achievement of developmental differentiation and maintenance of cell lineage identities [McNairn and Gilbert, 2003].

Expression of a retrovirus is controlled by cellular epigenetic regulation mechanisms. Indeed, a silent retrovirus stays silent after cell division, embryonic and postnatal development indicating that retrovirus silencing is heritable. The lack of expression of a silent retrovirus is not due to DNA sequence mutations. A silent retrovirus can be reactivated at least partially by drugs such as 5-bromodeoxyuridine (BrdU) [Bacheler et al., 1979] and the methylation inhibitor 5-azacytidine (5-AzaC) [Stewart et al., 1982] demonstrating that the integrated retrovirus is functional. The existence of variegated retrovirus vectors is another excellent demonstration of epigenetic regulation in retrovirus silencing. Cell clones with a variegated vector show intraclonal mosaicness with vector expression. Since the integrated retrovirus vector and its flanking endogenous genes are identical in different cells from the same clone, the variation of vector expression cannot be explained by DNA sequence differences. According to the definition of epigenetics, retrovirus silencing is an epigenetic phenomenon.

2. Epigenetic gene silencing background

It is well accepted that chromatin structure plays an important role in controlling and modulating eukaryotic gene expression [Wolffe and Guschin, 2000]. The basic unit of chromatin is the nucleosome composed of histone components with DNA wrapped around. In each nucleosome there is an octamer of histone H2A, H2B, H3 and H4. The histones forming the basic nucleosomal octamer are called core histones. About 145bp of DNA wraps 1.65 turns around the octamer. Linker DNA, the DNA between adjacent histone octamers, varies in length in different species and in metazoan is bound by linker histones such as histone H1.

Arrays of nucleosomes form 30nm diameter chromatin fibers, and linker histone H1 is involved in this process [Graziano et al., 1994]. Chromatin can be bound by non-histone proteins which are referred to as chromatin factors. Like linker histones the binding of chromatin factors induces special chromatin conformations. Heterochromatin, which was originally a term to define cytologically condensed regions of the genome throughout the cell cycle, is now widely used to refer to any silent chromatin domain. Correspondingly, euchromatin refers to active chromatin domains. Chromatin is the platform of gene transcription in eukaryotic cells.

Epigenetic silencing is achieved by establishing and maintaining a relatively inaccessible repressive chromatin domain [Grewal and Moazed, 2003; Wolffe and Matzke, 1999]. DNA methylation and other chromatin modifications induce a silent chromatin conformation by either recruiting repressive chromatin proteins or avoiding positive chromatin protein binding. These epigenetic chromatin modifications serve as heritable silencing marks to pass silent chromatin conformation through cell division [Moazed, 2001]. The inaccessibility of silent chromatin can be studied by its insensitivity to DNase digestion. Chromatin modifications can be studied by chromatin immunoprecipitation (ChIP) assays using modification specific antibodies [Crane-Robinson et al., 1999].

2.1. DNA methylation induced gene silencing

About 70-80% of the CpG dinucleotides are methylated at cytosine in mammalian cells. Early stage embryos of mammals experience a dramatic demethylation and remethylation [Santos et al., 2002]. These processes are believed to be essential in determining somatic DNA methylation patterns and critical for proper development of the embryo. Treatment with the methylation inhibitor 5-azacytidine or by genetically reducing overall genomic methylation levels through gene targeting of the methyltransferases can reactivate some gene expression. In fact, knockout of the mouse DNA methyltransferase Dnmt1 is embryonic lethal [Li et al., 1992]. These results show that DNA methylation plays a critical role in gene expression and development.

2.1.1. DNA methyltransferases

Three DNA methyltransferases have been identified in mammals (Figure 2A). Dnmt1 is the maintenance methylase with a preference for hemi-methylated DNA. It co-localizes with replication forks [Leonhardt et al., 1992]. The recent finding that Dnmt1 interacts with the clamping protein PCNA in the replication complex is consistent with the maintenance function of Dnmt1 [Iida et al., 2002]. Knocking down dnmt1 expression by antisense oligonucleotides triggers the intra-S-phase arrest of DNA replication [Milutinovic et al., 2003]. Dnmt3a and 3b are the two known de novo methylases [Okano et al., 1999; Xie et al., 1999]. Recent publications also demonstrate that Dnmt3a and 3b function in DNA methylation maintenance by assisting Dnmt1 [Liang et al., 2002].

Knocking out these two de novo methylases does not reduce the overall methylation levels in the genome. However, it does affect methylation on some genes such as endogenous and exogenous retrovirus, imprinting genes and satellite repeats. The dnmt3a knock out mice die 3 to 4 weeks after birth, while the dnmt3b knockout embryos do not develop further than

9.5 days after fertilization [Okano et al., 1999]. Dnmt3a and 3b have different isoforms. The existence of different isoforms in different cell types may determine the different methylation patterns on their genomic DNA. Dnmt2 has a domain homologous with other methylase catalyzing domains. No methylation activity by Dnmt2 has been observed [Okano et al., 1998], but *in vivo* antibody labeling does show Dnmt2 binding to genomic DNA [Liu et al., 2003]. Dnmt3L (dnmt3 like) shares homology with 3a and 3b, but lacks a functional catalytic domain. Dnmt3L assists other methylases in targeting maternal imprinted genes [Hata et al., 2002].

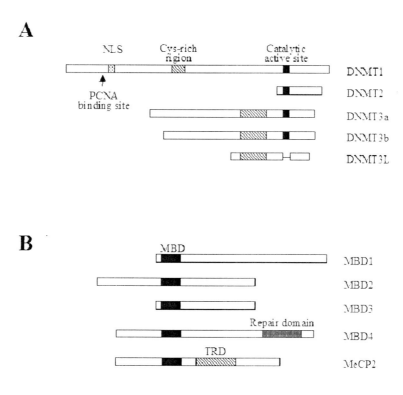

Figure 2. Mammalian DNA methyl-transferases and methylated DNA binding proteins. A). Mammalian DNA methyl-transferases. The methyl-transferase catalytic sites locate at the C-terminal. DNMT3L does not have a catalytic site. HDAC complex binds at the Cys-rich region. There is a NLS domain and a replication protein PCNA binding site at DNMT1 N-terminus. B). Mammalian methylated DNA binding proteins. MBD, methyl-CpG binding domain. The DNA repair domain of MBD4 locates at its C-terminus. MeCP2 has a transcription repression domain TRD [Bird and Wolffe, 1999].

3.1.2. Methylated DNA binding proteins and gene repression

DNA methylation can result in two modes of repression which are likely biologically relevant. First, methylation of DNA may interfere with trans-acting factors binding to the cognate DNA sequence. The transcriptional activator CpG binding protein (CGBP) serves as an example. This protein exhibits a unique binding specificity for DNA elements that contain unmethylated CpG motifs [Voo et al., 2000]. Knocking out CGBP is embryonic lethal demonstrating that this protein is crucial for early embryogenesis [Carlone and Skalnik, 2001]. The second mode of repression involves recruiting proteins to methyl-CpG (Figure 2B). The first methyl-CpG binding protein identified was MeCP2 [Lewis et al., 1992]. Dissection of MeCP2 revealed that an 85 amino acid methyl-CpG binding domain (MBD) can bind nonspecifically to one or more symmetrically methylated CpGs [Nan et al., 1993]. By searching expressed sequence tag (EST) databases, four other methyl-CpG binding proteins were identified named MBD1, MBD2, MBD3 and MBD4. MBD4 participates in DNA damage repair [Ballestar and Wolffe, 2001]. The other 4 MBD containing proteins have been implicated in methylation-dependent repression of transcription [Bird and Wolffe, 1999].

Nan et al [Nan et al., 1997] identified the transcriptional repression domain (TRD) in MeCP2 responsible for long-range repression *in vivo*. The TRD domain was later found to be associated with a corepressor complex containing sin3 and a histone deacetylase (HDAC) [Jones et al., 1998; Nan et al., 1998]. HDAC and other repressors were also found to associate with MBD1, MBD2 and MBD3 [Ballestar and Wolffe, 2001]. These findings established a direct causal relationship between DNA methylation and gene repression via chromatin modification. Recent publications further show that MeCP2 complexed with Sin3a is targeted directly to some promoters and represses gene expression [Chen et al., 2003; Martinowich et al., 2003; Stancheva et al., 2003]. However, lines of evidence suggest that other pathways may exist in MeCP2 induced gene repression. First, binding of MeCP2 can form a specific secondary condensed structure *in vitro* [Georgel et al., 2003]. Second, recent publications demonstrate that MeCP2 associates with histone methyltransferase *in vivo* and directs repressive histone Lys9 methylation [Fuks et al., 2003a; Fuks et al., 2003b].

2.2. Chromatin structure and gene silencing

Silent chromatin structure can be induced by histone covalent modification, or by linker histones or other accessory chromatin proteins. All histone proteins share similar structural characteristics. They have a globular domain essential for histone interaction with each other in nucleosomes [Wolffe and Guschin, 2000]. Flanking the globular domain, histones can have one or two non-structured tail domains that can be heavily covalently modified. Modification includes phosphorylation, acetylation, methylation, ADP ribosylation and ubiquitination [Berger, 2002]. Each of these modifications combined with their position on different histones has been reported to relate to different chromatin functions and chromatin structural alterations [Cheung et al., 2000]. In addition, findings of the interplay between these modifications on the same histone tail add another layer of complexity. Notably, histones are not the only proteins whose functions are regulated by post-translational modifications. Enzymes responsible for histone modification such as kinases are also involved in signaling transduction pathways. It was proposed that signaling pathways act directly on chromatin components to regulate different DNA-templated processes [Cheung et al., 2000]. Histone tail modifications and their combinatorial functions have been referred to as a Histone Code [Strahl and Allis, 2000].

2.2.1. Histone modification and gene silencing

Core histone deacetylation and methylation have been found to strongly correlate with gene silencing. Studies of bulk acetylation levels in yeast have shown that up to 13 of the 30 tail lysine residues in a histone octamer are acetylated [Roth et al., 2001]. Histone acetylation levels are maintained by the opposing actions of histone acetyltransferase (HAT) and histone deacetylase (HDAC) complexes [Reid et al., 2000; Vogelauer et al., 2000]. Both HATs and HDACs act as part of large complexes. There are multiple mechanisms by which deacetylation of histone tails might facilitate transcription silencing. Deacetylation may stabilize the interaction between histones and DNA by alteration of the N-terminal charge; or may facilitate the internucleosomal interaction via the histone tail; or may recruit additional chromatin accessory proteins [Narlikar et al., 2002]. Also, deacetylation of histone tails may facilitate other modifications on the same histone tail which may induce further chromatin alteration.

Histone lysine methylation occurs on lysine residues 4, 9, 27 and 36 in H3, position 20 in H4 and also the H1 amino terminus. Suv39 is the first histone methyltransferase (HMTase) to be identified. Identification of the HMTase catalytic domain (Suv39-E(z)-Trithorax domain, SET domain) led to the identification of more than 70 gene sequences containing SET domain in mammals. Suv39h, G9a and Ezh2 are involved in histone H3 Lys9 and Lys27 methylation [Cao et al., 2002; Czermin et al., 2002; Rea et al., 2000; Tachibana et al., 2001]. Suv39h induced histone H3 Lys9 methylation can be bound by HP1 and induce heterochromatin [Peters et al., 2001]. Suv39h is also reported to be involved in repression of euchromatic genes [Nielsen et al., 2001]. Lys27 tri-methylation is observed in X-inactivation and bound by PcG proteins [Cao et al., 2002]. Histone H3 Lys4 methylation is induced by another SET protein MLL and associates with gene expression [Milne et al., 2002]. Interestingly, both Ezh2 and MLL are polycomb/trithrox group (PcG/trxG) proteins. PcG/trxG are involved in epigenetic cellular memory in *Drosophila* [Pirrotta, 1998]. These findings suggest that histone H3 Lys9 and Lys4 tri-methylation may serve as signals for eukaryotic epigenetic regulation memory.

2.2.2. Accessory chromatin proteins and gene silencing

In addition to nucleosomes, the chromatin fiber contains a diversity of other accessory proteins including linker histone and other non-histone proteins. The binding of linker histone H1 is dynamic [Lever et al., 2000; Misteli et al., 2000]. The displacement of H1 is modulated by cdk2 mediated phosphorylation [Bhattacharjee et al., 2001; Horn et al., 2002]. The binding of linker histone H1 is believed to form a closed chromatin conformation [Karymov et al., 2001] and induce gene silencing on some genes but not all [Shen and Gorovsky, 1996].

Non-histone chromatin accessory proteins are the proteins present in some chromatin structures, which are not essential to form a functional chromatin structure. This includes methylated DNA binding proteins (MBDs), heterochromatin protein 1 (HP1) [Eissenberg and Elgin, 2000], silencing information regulator (Sir) [Shore, 2000], high mobility group (HMG) proteins [Ner and Travers, 1994] and PcG/TrxG proteins etc. The binding of these factors can alter chromatin structure. Some chromatin factors alter chromatin structure via histone tail covalent modification. For example, PcG protein Ezh2 catalyzes histone H3 Lysine27 tri-methylation [Czermin et al., 2002]. Others can form higher order chromatin structures like linker H1, HP1 [Eissenberg and Elgin, 2000] and PcG proteins [Sewalt et al., 2002]. A common character of most chromatin accessory proteins is their ability to form polymers which can spread a specific chromatin conformation into and subsequently silence flanking DNA sequences.

2.3. Gene silencing network

Broad interplay among different chromatin alterations has been reported. Interplay can happen between the same levels of chromatin alterations. For example, MeCP2 was reported to replace linker histone H1 *in vitro* [Nan et al., 1997]. Lys9 deacetylation is proposed as a prerequisite for methylation at the same lysine residual [Cheung et al., 2000]. However, often the interplay is between different chromatin alteration levels. Histone tail modification such as H3 Lys9 methylation determines chromatin accessory protein binding. MeCP2 bound on methylated DNA can induce histone H3 deacetylation and methylation [Fuks et al., 2003b]. Also, H3 methylation is reported to direct DNA methylation in yeast [Schramke and Allshire, 2003] and plants [Jackson et al., 2002]. Chromatin modifications such as DNA methylation and histone modifications can be recognized by specific binding proteins. The binding proteins can subsequently recruit other chromatin modification enzymes to the same gene. As a result multiple chromatin modifications and multiple chromatin alterations co-exist on the same gene to enforce chromatin structures, be it condensed or open. It is reasonable to hypothesize that DNA methylation, histone modifications, and chromatin factor binding are all parts of a gene repression network. They function separately and cooperatively to achieve an inaccessible chromatin conformation.

2.4. Variegated epigenetic silencing

Variegated epigenetic silencing is observed in *Drosophila*, yeast and transgenic mice and is designated as position effect variegation (PEV). The prototype PEV phenomenon was observed in *Drosophila*. When a normally active euchromatic gene is translocated into the boundary between heterochromatin and euchromatin, its expression is shut down in a portion of the cells due to the spreading of condensed heterochromatin into the translocated gene. PEV of the eye color *white* gene results in the eye color mosaicness in *Drosophilia*. Massive genetic screens led to the identification of a large amount of PEV modifier genes in *Drosophila* [Schotta et al., 2002]. Among them, some can induce chromatin modification and structural alteration [Schotta et al., 2002].

PEV is also observed in transgenic mice. Transgene expression in mouse lines with multicopy transgenes does not correlate with the number of integrated transgene copies indicating an important role for integration sites. Transgene "copy number independent and position dependent" expression can be avoided by inclusion of locus control regions (LCR). LCRs are gene regulatory elements in mammals and birds that can overcome the repressive effects associated with heterochromatic transgene locations to promote position-independent and copy number-dependent transgene expression [Kioussis and Festenstein, 1997]. Transgenes with partially deleted LCRs located at the edge of centromeric heterochromatin regions are subject to PEV [Festenstein et al., 1996; Milot et al., 1996]. Using these PEV mouse lines, Milot and others have shown that PEV is controlled by the balance of positive transcription factors (Sp1 and EKLF) and repressive chromatin modifiers (Suv39H1, HP1, and PcG proteins) [Festenstein et al., 1999; Lundgren et al., 2000; McMorrow et al., 2000]. Interestingly, while most of the PEV in transgenic mice occurs when transgenes are located in heterochromatin, a recent paper demonstrates that PEV also can be established in non-centromeric regions [Ayyanathan et al., 2003].

3. Model Systems Used In Retrovirus Silencing Studies

From the first retrovirus silencing experiment done over 20 years ago, different model systems have been used. In general the model systems used for retrovirus silencing can be categorized into two groups: infection models and transfection models. In infection models, retrovirus or retrovirus vectors are infected into primitive cell types. In transfection models, retrovirus DNA sequences with or without modifications are introduced into different cell types. Both of these models have provided useful information on retrovirus silencing. Understanding the advantages and disadvantages of these systems is crucial to compare the data from different publications. The proper usage of retrovirus silencing systems is also important for the development of silencing-resistant retrovirus vectors.

3.1. Infection models

In the infection models, retrovirus or retrovirus vectors are infected into preimplantation embryos, EC, ES or HSC. Comparison of retrovirus vector expression in primitive cells and mature cells is commonly used to determine retrovirus silencing effects. The existence of provirus DNA is used to determine successful viral infection. When wildtype retrovirus is used, infectious viral particles and viral protein expression are used to detect retrovirus expression. Expression of retrovirus vectors is detected by the expression of reporter genes. Because retrovirus vector infected cells cannot make infectious retrovirus vectors, it can avoid the virus spread problem associated with wildtype retrovirus infection. The existence of easily detectable reporter genes gives retrovirus vectors another advantage. Retrovirus vector infection models provide a unique opportunity to study different types of retrovirus silencing phenomena and their mechanisms. An infection model is also important to evaluate novel silencing-resistant retrovirus vector design.

Multiple copy provirus integration is a potential problem in infection models. The existence of expressing retrovirus vector can mask silent vectors in the same cell. The silent retrovirus vector transduced cells are also mixed with an excess of untransduced cells. The isolation and identification of single copy vector transduced cell lines are crucial to retrovirus silencing study. The use of *in vitro* cultured primitive cells facilitates the isolation and identification of silent retrovirus. The existence of homologous endogenous retrovirus in the mouse genome is another potential problem. It makes the determination of viral integration difficult. This problem can be avoided by careful design of retrovirus vectors.

Recently, HSC were used as model systems mainly because of their potential use in blood disease gene therapy. Research on HSC is always hampered by the lack of identity of HSC cells [Trevisan and Iscove, 1995]. Because the absolute purification of HSC is not possible, it is difficult to distinguish retrovirus expression in transduced HSC cells from other progenitor cells. One way to avoid this problem is serial transplantation. Since only HSC cells can survive after serial transplantation, the expression of the retrovirus vectors has to derive from HSC cells [Challita and Kohn, 1994].

3.2. Transfection models

To study the involvement of DNA methylation in retrovirus silencing, two different transfection systems were introduced. M. Lorincz transfected *in vitro* methylated or unmethylated retrovirus sequences into a specific integration site in murine erythroleukemia (MEL) cells [Lorincz et al., 2001; Lorincz et al., 2002]. While this system can clearly determine whether DNA methylation functions in retrovirus silencing, the disadvantage is that the result might heavily depend on the integration site being used. Transgenic *Drosophila* also can be used to investigate the involvement of DNA methylation in retrovirus silencing. *Drosophila* was long believed to be a methylation-free system [Urieli-Shoval et al., 1982]. D. Pannell in our laboratory established that retrovirus sequences function as silencers in transgenic *Drosophila* suggesting that retrovirus silencing can be established independent of DNA methylation [Pannell et al., 2000]. However, a small amount of DNA methylation is detected in *Drosophila* especially in early embryos [Lyko et al., 2000]. The function of this DNA methylation is not yet clear. Nevertheless, the DNA methylation in *Drosophila* is not likely the same as in mammals, because the methylase being used is homologous to Dnmt2 [Hung et al., 1999] while Dnmt2 is not functional as a methylase in mammals [Okano et al., 1998]. The use of these two models has provided great information on whether and how DNA methylation is involved in retrovirus silencing.

Transfection models were also used to identify and modify silencer elements in retrovirus vectors. When a retrovirus sequence was linked to an LCR β-globin reporter gene and microinjected into fertilized mouse eggs, silencing of the reporter gene by the retrovirus sequence was detected in fetal liver [McCune and Townes, 1994; Osborne et al., 1999]. Transgene DNA and its expression were evaluated in each embryo. The silencing effect was evaluated by the percentage of expressing embryos and their expression levels. Since transgene expression suffers from PEV, a strong reporter gene that can promote position independent transgene expression is important to this model, and therefore a human LCR β-globin cassette was used as the reporter gene for retrovirus silencers. The human β-globin LCR is composed of four DNase I-hypersensitive sites all of which are required for full LCR activity [Pasceri et al., 1998]. The reporter cassette we used contains a 3.0-kb LCR(5'HS2 to 5'HS4) linked to the human β-globin transgene and directs 16 to 71% expression at all integration sites [Ellis et al., 1997]. The transgenic mouse model is very useful for evaluation of modifications to retrovirus vector silencer elements and development of silencing resistant retrovirus vectors.

4. Retrovirus Vector Silencing Mechanisms

4.1. Genome Defence Hypothesis

During the course of evolution, cells have been exposed to foreign DNAs. Intragenomic parasites are one of the important pathways for cellular genomes to obtain new genes. But integration of intragenomic parasites can cause endogenous gene damage and misregulation, so is potentially harmful. Genome defence systems may have developed during evolution to ensure genome integrity [Doerfler, 1991]. The genome defense hypothesis contends that cytosine methylation arose in mammals to restrict expression of intragenomic parasites [Walsh and Bestor, 1999]. Evidence supporting the genome defense hypothesis stems from the finding that the LTRs of retrotransposable elements such as L1s, IAPs, and endogenous retroviruses are all heavily methylated at CpG dinucleotides [Yoder et al., 1997a; Yoder et al., 1997b]. Further evidence supporting a role for methylation in genome defense comes from the finding that the IAP class of endogenous retrovirus becomes reactivated in ES cells that are null for the maintenance methyltransferase Dnmt1 [Walsh et al., 1998]. Notably DNA methylation is also involved in the restriction-modification system of bacterial defense function indicating that DNA methylation is an old player in cell defense [Bestor, 1990].

4.2. DNA methylation and retrovirus silencing

4.2.1. Functional role of DNA methylation in retrovirus silencing

Silencing of retrovirus is often accompanied by high density cytosine methylation [Jahner et al., 1982; Stewart et al., 1982]. The methylation inhibiting drug 5-azacytidine (5-AzaC) has been used to reactivate silent provirus in EC cells [Stewart et al., 1982]. The Jaenisch laboratory demonstrated that *in vitro* methylated retrovirus DNA is not infectious in cells, but treatment of the recipient cells with 5-AzaC reactivated infectious virus [Simon et al., 1983]. A functional role of DNA methylation in retrovirus silencing and extinction has been demonstrated [Cherry et al., 2000; Lorincz et al., 2000; Lorincz et al., 2001]. Recently Swindle et al [Swindle et al., 2004] also showed a causal role of DNA methylation in establishment and maintenance of retrovirus silencing by mutating the LTR promoter region CpGs.

It is proposed that the binding of MBD proteins on methylated DNA recruits HDACs and subsequently represses gene expression [Ballestar and Wolffe, 2001; Jones et al., 1998; Nan et al., 1998]. MeCP2 is recruited to silent retrovirus sequence [Lorincz et al., 2001; Yao, 2004]. However, no reactivation was observed by the HDAC inhibitor TSA or sodium butyrate alone in silent ES cells [Yao, 2004]. Clearly mechanisms other than histone deacetylation exist in the DNA methylation dependent retrovirus silencing pathway.

4.2.2. DNA methylation independent pathway of retrovirus silencing

While there is data supporting a causal role of DNA methylation in retrovirus silencing, several lines of data suggest other mechanisms may also exist. First, 5-AzaC reactivation of silent retrovirus is only partial. This suggests that other methylation-independent mechanisms are actively silencing some of retroviruses in these cells. Second, retrovirus silencing is established much earlier than DNA methylation. Silencing occurs in EC cells 2 days post-infection whereas methylation is not detectable until 8-16 days [Gautsch and Wilson, 1983; Niwa et al., 1983]. Third, retrovirus silencing can be established in *Drosophila*. Because *Drosophila* is a DNA methylation free environment, this result suggests that DNA methylation is not essential for retrovirus silencing [Pannell et al., 2000]. Fourth, among the identified silencers in retrovirus LTR, the promoter is the only CpG-rich silencer. DNA methylation induced retrovirus silencing cannot account for the other silencers function.

Dnmt3a and 3b are the only de novo methylases known to methylate exogenous transduced retrovirus. Identification of silent retrovirus in dnmt3ab knockout ES cells is the best way to test the existence of DNA methylation independent retrovirus silencing pathway. In deed, silent single copy retrovirus vector transduced dnmt3ab-/- ES cell clones were identified in our lab. DNA methylation sensitive digestion confirmed no DNA methylation on the integrated retrovirus [Yao, 2004], demonstrating the existence of a DNA methylation independent retrovirus silencing pathway.

4.2.3. Relationship between DNA methylation dependent and independent pathways

Recently, multiple pathways functioning stepwise in retrovirus silencing have been proposed. MoMLV vector infected MEL cells that initially expressed were sorted and silencing was examined over time. It was found that an initial extinction event is reversible by the HDAC inhibitor trichostatin A (TSA). At later time points, reactivation of expression required 5-AzaC in conjunction with trichostatin A, suggesting that methylation is a secondary step associated with maintenance of silencing [Lorincz et al., 2000; Lorincz et al., 2002]. By studying retrovirus infected ES cell long-term culture extinction, S. Cherry also proposed that there are DNA-methylation independent pathways at early stages and dependent pathways at later stages in retrovirus silencing [Cherry et al., 2000]. However, retrovirus silencing occurs in *do novo* methylase null ES cells [Yao, 2004]. Therefore, both DNA methylation dependent and independent pathways are capable of maintaining retrovirus silencing. We propose that DNA methylation dependent and independent pathways function in parallel in gene repression.

4.3. Chromatin conformation in retrovirus silencing

Retrovirus provirus is integrated into the host genome and inherited with other endogenous genes [Breindl et al., 1979]. Epigenetic mechanisms such as histone modification and chromatin accessory protein binding may therefore also function on integrated provirus DNA. In 1979, Breindl and Jaenisch published that the chromatin conformation of transduced retrovirus is altered in the permissive and non-permissive tissue of the same mouse line by comparing their sensitivity to DNase digestion. In the non-permissive tissue in which the infected retrovirus is silent, the provirus is more resistant to DNase I digestion suggesting a condensed conformation [Breindl and Jaenisch, 1979]. DNase I hypersensitive site alteration was also observed in an endogenous allele mutated by Mo-MuLV insertion [Breindl et al., 1984].

Retrovirus sequence can silence the linked human LCR β-globin transgene in transgenic mice. Using ChIP assay, we have shown that the retrovirus silenced transgene is marked by silent chromatin characterized by histone H3 deacetylation and linker histone H1 [Pannell et al., 2000]. These results demonstrate that histone modifications are involved in retrovirus silencing. A similar silent chromatin is formed on the silent retrovirus vectors in genuine infected ES cells as well as the silenced retrovirus in variegated ES cells [Yao, 2004]. As in wildtype ES cells, silent retrovirus vectors in *dnmt3ab-/-* cells are also marked by histone H3 deacetylation and linker histone H1 binding [Yao, 2004]. The existence of similar chromatin conformation on silent retrovirus regardless of DNA methylation shows that silent chromatin is a universal mark for retrovirus silencing.

No reactivation was observed by TSA treatment on retrovirus silenced transgene in transgenic mice [Pannell et al., 2000] and silenced retrovirus in transduced ES cells [Yao, 2004]. TSA treatment can increase the acetylation level of silenced transgene in transgenic mice, however TSA treatment cannot remove the linker histone H1 (unpublished data). These results suggest an important role for histone H1 in maintaining retrovirus silencing. The binding of histone H1 in silent *dnmt3ab-/-* cells is more abundant than in wildtype ES cells [Yao, 2004]. Since MeCP2 can replace histone H1 in binding linker DNA [Nan et al., 1997], we propose there is a compensatory competition between H1 and MeCP2 binding. When MeCP2 cannot bind, histone H1 will take over to maintain silent chromatin. This dynamic interplay of different pathways directs silent chromatin formation and maintenance.

5. Retrovirus Silencing Insulation

5.1. Retrovirus vectors that resist silencing

The existence of retrovirus silencing in stem cells indicates the need to develop silencing-resistant retrovirus vectors. Development of such retrovirus vectors started with the isolation of EC cell permissive retrovirus strains and continued with the identification and removal of silencer elements from retrovirus vectors. Self-inactivating (SIN) retrovirus vectors are vectors with a deletion in 3'LTR promoter region so that there are no functional promoters in any of the provirus LTRs after vector transduction. Although SIN retrovirus vectors were originally developed to improve vector safety, the extreme deletion of the retrovirus sequences in SIN vectors also reduces retrovirus silencing. Combining these efforts, many retrovirus vectors have been developed for stem cell gene transfer and gene therapy.

The identification and characterization of multiple silencer elements in retrovirus vectors paved the way for the construction of numerous modified vectors that lack these sequences. Silencer elements are DNA binding sites for trans-acting factors that directly or indirectly reduce transcription at promoters. At least four separate silencer elements located in the LTRs and the adjacent primer binding site (PBS) have been identified in retrovirus vectors. The LTR promoter is CpG rich serving as a potential silencer [Osborne et al., 1999; Swindle et al., 2004]. The Negative Control Region (NCR) was identified in the upstream region of the LTR which reduces virus expression [Flanagan et al., 1989]. Mutations in the direct repeat (DR) of the LTR enhancer were found to increase expression in stem cells [Hilberg et al., 1987]. The groups of Jaenisch and Goff found mutant PBS sites that increased expression from the LTR [Barklis et al., 1986; Colicelli and Goff, 1986]. Several negative trans-acting factors had been found to bind these silencer elements. Specifically, the multi-functional transcriptional regulator YY-1 binds to NCR [Flanagan et al., 1992], six distinct nuclear factors bind to each of the DRs [Speck and Baltimore, 1987], and the PBS is bound by factor A [Petersen et al., 1991]. In addition, the embryonic LTR-binding protein (ELP) [Tsukiyama and Niwa, 1992] was found to bind between the NCR and DR [Tsukiyama et al., 1989]. It has been shown that no single silencer element is sufficient to induce complete silencing [Osborne et al., 1999], suggesting that silencer elements additively increase the probability of silencing via multiple mechanisms.

Mo-MuLV is one of the earliest retrovirus isolated and studied. Given its well understood biology and its ability to efficiently infect a wide range of cells, Mo-MuLV has been widely used to derive retrovirus vectors. One problem for wildtype Mo-MuLV vectors is they are not permissive in ES or EC cells because of the poor functionality of Mo-MuLV LTR enhancer in these cells [Tsukiyama et al., 1989]. PCMV is a mutant form of myeloproliferative sarcoma virus (MPSV) containing a deletion of one of the enhancer DRs, as well as a mutation in the ELP binding site and a point mutation that introduces an Sp1 binding site [Hilberg et al., 1987]. Although the PCMV enhancer is functional in both EC and ES cells, PCMV derived vectors are still restricted in ES cells [Grez et al., 1990]. Combination of the PCMV LTR with a PBS from an integration-defective Mo-MuLV mutant dl587rev [Colicelli and Goff, 1987] which does not bind factor A, yields the murine embryonic stem cell virus (MESV) [Grez et al., 1990]. Hawley et al further refined the MESV vector to increase titers by including an extended packaging signal from the LN vector and an upstream gag sequence from Moloney murine sarcoma virus, (MoMSV) resulting in MSCV [Hawley, 1994]. MSCV retains silencer elements such as the NCR, one of the DRs, and the CpG rich promoter.

Substitution of the MoMLV enhancer has been another approach to improve retrovirus vector expression in primitive cells. The MPSV (myeloproliferative sarcoma virus) enhancer had been shown to have increased expression in EC cells [Hilberg et al., 1987]. Substitution of the Mo-MuLV LTR with the MPSV LTR in conjunction with the dl587rev PBS yielded the MD (MPSV, dl587rev) vector [Challita et al., 1995]. Unfortunately, the expression from the MD vector did not significantly increase. However, the MND (MPSV, NCR, dl587rev) vector derived from a deletion of the NCR in the MD vector did show substantial improvement with expression in 43% of infected EC cells [Challita et al., 1995]. The MND vector also showed significantly increased expression in murine hematopoietic stem cells (HSCs) [Robbins et al., 1998].

Finally, SIN retrovirus vectors have steadily gained popularity due to the decreased probability that these vectors will undergo recombination leading to the generation of a rescued infectious virus. The first Mo-MuLV-based SIN retrovirus vector used a 299bp deletion in the 3'LTR that removes most of the DR and the promoter, but retains the NCR and wild-type PBS [Yu et al., 1986]. More recently the HSC1 vector was constructed in our laboratory by deletion of the entire NCR, DR, and part of the CpG rich promoter sequence in MSCV which retains the mutant PBS. HSC1 vector directs neo expression in 71% of transduced EC cells, offering a further improvement still [Osborne et al., 1999]. The HSC1 vector is particularly attractive both for its ability to express in non-permissive environments and its SIN properties.

SIN-Lentivirus vectors were created for safety reasons and may express better in primitive cell types due to the deletion of potential silencer sequences from the LTRs [Miyoshi et al., 1998]. Indeed, SIN-Lentivirus vector has been shown to transduce more efficiently into a broad range of cell types with higher expression levels compared with vectors with intact LTRs [Miyoshi et al., 1998]. Notably, the experience and knowledge gained in developing retrovirus vectors are well transferred into Lentivirus vector development.

In summary, progressive deletion or mutation of silencer sequences has lead to the development of retroviral vectors that have an increased probability of expression in primitive cell types. However, none of the current vectors are able to express at all integration sites despite mutations in all known retroviral silencer elements, suggesting that novel silencer elements remain to be discovered and may reside in the essential sequences of retrovirus vectors. In this consideration, insulation of the retrovirus silencer elements should be the next step in development of silencing resistant vectors.

5.2. Insulator elements

The eukaryotic nucleus is organized into active and inactive domains [Weintraub and Groudine, 1976]. Within each chromosomal domain, each gene is embedded within a chromosomal environment of other DNA sequences that have the potential to affect its expression. Boundary elements such as insulators are needed to keep different domains and genes functioning separately. Insulators are defined as DNA elements located between different functional chromosomal domains that keep each of these domains functioning properly. In practice, insulators are defined by two assays: Enhancer Effect Blocking Assay [Kellum and Schedl, 1991] and Position Effect Protection Assay [Kellum and Schedl, 1992] (Figure 3A). Insulators can block the enhancing effect of an enhancer on a promoter. Transgenes in different integration sites suffer from PEV. Flanking transgenes with insulators can block position effects and promote position-independent transgene expression. Insulator elements themselves should have no enhancer, silencer or promoter activity. In other words, insulator elements should be neutral to make sure the blocking effect observed in these two assays is the result of true insulation. Insulator elements have silencer blocking activity. Otte and colleagues showed that insulators block silencing effects of LexA silencing factor fusion proteins recruited to episomal reporter genes in human cells [van der Vlag et al., 2000]. Insulator silencer blocking activity was also tested in transgenic *Drosophila* [Barolo and Levine, 1997; Cai and Levine, 1995]. Insulator elements are found in *Drosophila* (*gypsy*, scs/scs', Fab-7, Fab-8, etc.) yeast (HMR, STAR etc.), sea urchin (sns), birds (cHS4) and mammals (H19/Ig2f, BEAD-1, HS5, etc.) [Bell and Felsenfeld, 1999]. Among them, chicken HS4 (cHS4), *Drosophila gypsy* and Scs are three well studied insulator elements.

Insulator elements were first discovered in *Drosophilia*. Scs/Scs' (special chromatin structures) insulators are located at the boundaries of the heat-shock *hsp70* gene and protect it from stimulation by neighboring genes [Udvardy et al., 1985]. These elements were shown to protect white transgenes against chromosomal position effects to produce uniform eye color [Kellum and Schedl, 1991]. Later the same group also showed that scs/scs' can block enhancer effects [Kellum and Schedl, 1992]. BEAF-32A and BEAF-32B (a boundary-element-associated factor of 32kDa) were found to bind to scs' [Hart et al., 1997; Zhao et al., 1995]. Zest-white-5 (Zw-5) binds to scs insulator [Gaszner et al., 1999]. BEAF was found to locate at hundreds of interbands and many puff boundaries on polytene chromosomes[Zhao et al., 1995].

Gypsy insulator is another *Drosophila* insulator that has been extensively studied. It was originally found in the 5' non-translated region of *Drosophila gypsy* retrotransposon [Geyer and Corces, 1992]. Insertion of the *gypsy* retrotransposon in the yellow gene blocks enhancers located upstream of the insertion site causing abnormal eye pigmentation. A 430-bp fragment of the 5' non-translated region was found to be responsible for this blocking. *Gypsy* insulator was also reported to protect a DNA replication origin from position effects [Lu and Tower, 1997] and to block polycomb group (PcG) protein induced gene repression [Mallin et al., 1998]. Interestingly, when multiple *gypsy* insulators were placed between an enhancer and promoter, or the enhancer was flanked with two *gypsy* insulators no insulation was observed [Cai and Shen, 2001; Melnikova et al., 2002; Muravyova et al., 2001]. Su(Hw) (Suppressor Hairy-wing) protein is required for *gypsy* insulator enhancer-blocking activity in *Drosophila*, and the *mod(mdg4)* gene is also involved [Gause et al., 2001; Gdula et al., 1996; Ghosh et al., 2001]. These two proteins direct *gypsy* insulator DNA to the nuclear periphery [Gerasimova et al., 2000]. No Su(Hw) homologue has been found in mammalian cells, but *gypsy* insulator was found to be bound by mammalian nuclear matrix proteins and function as a matrix attachment region (MAR) element [Nabirochkin et al., 1998]. Most recently the *gypsy* insulator was also reported to serve as a MAR in *Drosophila* [Byrd and Corces, 2003]. MAR elements are binding sites for nuclear scaffold proteins *in vitro* and are proposed to attach chromatin to the nuclear matrix *in vivo* [Dickinson et al., 1992]. It is proposed that some MAR elements can shield transgenes from the influence of flanking genes [Allen et al., 2000; Bonifer et al., 1994].

The first and the best-characterized vertebrate insulator element is the cHS4 insulator of the chicken β-globin gene (Figure 3B). The β-globin locus in chicken erythrocytes contains a 33-kb domain of open chromatin and a 16-kb stretch of heterochromatin [Litt et al., 2001a; Litt et al., 2001b]. Upstream of this 16-kb heterochromatin domain is the folate receptor gene which is regulated distinctly from that of globin genes [Prioleau et al., 1999]. The 1.2kb cHS4 insulator is located at the boundary between the active globin domain and the heterochromatin domain. cHS4 insulator showed position effect protection activity [Chung et al., 1993] and enhancer blocking activity [Chung et al., 1997]. It blocks the spreading of histone deacetylation from heterochromatin but not DNA methylation [Mutskov et al., 2002]. A 250-bp CpG island that contains the constitutive DNase I hypersensitive site was found to retain most of the insulating activity. This 250-bp core element is used as a dimer to achieve full insulation [Chung et al., 1997]. Further dissection of the 250-bp core element found that only the footprint II bound by CTCF is required for enhancer blocking activity [Bell et al., 1999]. CTCF is a ubiquitous zinc-finger DNA-binding protein which recognizes multiple DNA sequences [Burcin et al., 1997; Klenova et al., 1998]. CTCF is involved in multiple functions such as gene silencing, gene activation, X-inactivation and insulator activity [Lutz et al., 2000]. Position effect protecting activity of the cHS4 core element does not require CTCF binding and resides in the other binding sites in the core element [Recillas-Targa et al., 2002]. The proteins responsible for position effect protection are not known.

5.3. Insulation of retrovirus and Lentivirus silencing

Expression of integrated retrovirus may be influenced by the flanking chromosomal environment of the integration site [Verma and Somia, 1997]. On the other hand, insertion of retrovirus also can induce insertional gene activation or repression [Breindl et al., 1984]. All retrovirus vectors contain LTRs and *gag* sequences that harbor known [Challita et al., 1995] and unidentified [Osborne et al., 1999] silencers. These elements can silence the transgene harbored in the retrovirus vector and potentially genomic genes flanking the integration site. Similarly, constant high expression of the retrovirus vector can activate flanking genes. Insulators are *cis*-acting elements and theoretically can be used to block retrovirus silencing

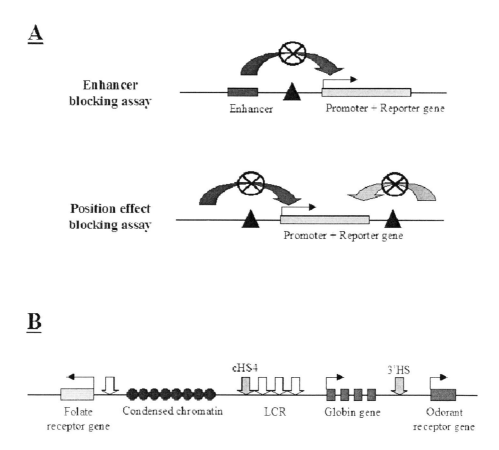

Figure 3. Insulator element. A. Two assays used to define insulator elements. In the enhancer blocking assay, the insulator element (black triangle) located between the enhancer and promoter will block the enhancer effect. In the position effect blocking assay, flanking the transgene with the insulator elements will protect the transgene from position effects from flanking endogenous genes. B, location of chicken HS4 insulator in the globin gene locus. cHS4 and 3'HS are two identified insulator elements functioning as boundary elements between different chromatin domains [Recillas-Targa et al., 2002]. See text for detail.

spread and protect a transgene harbored inside a retrovirus vector. In addition, insulator elements also can be used to block silencing or activating effects of retrovirus sequences and protect the genes flanking the integration sites.

The monomer 1.2-kb cHS4 insulator has been used in retrovirus and Lentivirus vectors with limited success. Insertion of cHS4 into a Mo-MuLV construct 3'LTR can be faithfully duplicated into two LTRs after retroviral integration. The insulated retrovirus promotes an increased probability of expression at random chromosomal integration sites in MEL cells. Unfortunately, improved reporter gene eGFP expression was not observed when used to infect ES cells [Rivella et al., 2000]. Similar retrovirus vectors based on the MSCV vector were constructed by D. Emery [Emery et al., 2000]. cHS4 in one orientation in MSCV LTRs supports high percentage GFP positive cells and high GFP expression level in both 3T3 and bone marrow derived blood cells. However extinction of retrovirus expression was observed in long-term reconstituted mice. Further experiments showed that cHS4 insulators in the LTRs dramatically decrease gene expression from an internal pgk promoter. In addition, severe differentiation extinction was observed regardless of the existence of cHS4 insulator [Yannaki et al., 2002]. At the same time, the same vector harboring a γ-globin cassette was able to successfully reduce gene silencing [Emery et al., 2002]. Notably, the γ-globin expression cassette used in this vector has its own enhancer. Similarly, cHS4 also failed to protect Lentivirus vector when located in LTRs in transduced CD34+ blood cells [Ramezani et al., 2003]. However, when the insertion of cHS4 in LTRs was combined with insertion of a matrix attachment region (MAR) element, higher and uniform gene expression was achieved [Ramezani and Hawley, 2003]. The same vector was also reported to support better gene expression in human ES cells although long term culture extinction was not avoided [Ma et al., 2003].

Use of insulators in retrovirus or Lentivirus vectors is mostly unsuccessful due to the lack of knowledge of retrovirus silencer blocking. Current insulator assays define the enhancer blocking activity and position effect protection activity of insulator elements. However, retrovirus silencer blocking activity is different from these two activities. Retrovirus silencing is a negative effect on the transgene from retrovirus sequences. Blocking a retrovirus silencer is not the same as blocking enhancer effects. Also, silencer blocking is not necessarily equal to position effect protection. In retrovirus vectors, the transgene is flanked by retrovirus silencers from both the 5' and 3'LTR. Retrovirus silencers may affect the transgene more than the flanking genomic DNA sequences simply because they are closer to the transgene. Our and other reports all show that blocking position effects by flanking retrovirus vectors with insulators is not sufficient to avoid silencing [Emery et al., 2000; Rivella et al., 2000; Yao et al., 2003]. An assay specific for retrovirus silencer blocking is needed to identify insulator elements suitable to be used in retrovirus vectors. In our work, an LCR β-globin expression cassette is used as a reporter transgene to evaluate the blocking of retrovirus silencer effects in transgenic mouse fetal liver cells [Yao et al., 2003]. Retrovirus sequences can silence this LCR β-globin transgene when linked directly [Osborne et al., 1999; Pannell et al., 2000]. Insulators with retrovirus silencer blocking activity will be able to protect transgene expression when inserted between the transgene and retrovirus sequence. Using this assay we screened different insulator elements and found that cHS4 has the ability to block retrovirus silencers [Yao et al., 2003]. The identification of retrovirus silencer blocking insulator elements is important to the design of insulated retrovirus vectors to avoid retrovirus silencing.

Using our retrovirus silencer blocking assay, we also showed retrovirus silencer blocking activity is independent of CTCF binding [Yao et al., 2003]. CTCF binding is the common feature for vertebrate insulator element enhancer blocking activities [Bell et al., 1999]. Therefore, this result further supports retrovirus silencer blocking activity is different from enhancer blocking activity. When the cHS4 dimer core insulator is used to flank the LCR β-globin reporter gene, full levels of expression were observed in the transgenic mice [Yao et al., 2003]. This result suggests the transgene in a retrovirus vector needs to be flanked by insulators to achieve full protection. However, flanking the reporter gene in retrovirus vectors with the cHS4 dimer core insulator failed to produce high titer virus suggesting another non-homologous insulator is needed to combine with cHS4 [Yao et al., 2003].

No silencer blocking activity was observed with *gypsy* and Scs insulator. However the *gypsy* insulator was observed to increase transgene expression when located in the retrovirus LTRs. cHS4, on the other hand, does not increase transgene expression in the same configuration. This result indicates that the *gypsy* insulator does not increase transgene expression by blocking retrovirus silencers [Yao et al., 2003]. *Gypsy* was reported to function as a MAR element in both *Drosophila* [Byrd and Corces, 2003] and mammalian cells [Nabirochkin et al., 1998]. The increase of transgene expression by *gypsy* in retrovirus vectors may be due to its ability to tether the transgene to the nuclear matrix. Regardless of the mechanism, the increase of transgene expression by *gypsy* insulator can be used to design high expressing retrovirus vectors.

An ideal insulated retrovirus vector would be able to protect both the internal transgene and the integration site flanking endogenous genes. Currently all the insulated retrovirus vectors use insulators located in LTRs and aim to block position effects from the flanking sequences and to prevent induction of insertional activation. However, some of the retrovirus silencers especially those located in 5'LTR and *gag* sequences are left between the two insulators and adjacent to the transgene. To completely protect the transgene, two different insulators should be used, one located in the U3 region of LTRs, the other between 5'LTR-PBS and the internal transgene. In this configuration, the transgene will be flanked by two insulators to achieve high expression and the flanking genomic genes will also be partially insulated from the integrated retrovirus vector.

6. Retrovirus Silencing Model

Although retrovirus vector silencing has long been documented, there is still argument about whether retrovirus silencing is solely due to position effects. Although the integration site flanking chromatin may be involved in the decision, the silencing of retrovirus vectors is mainly due to effects induced by the silencer elements in retrovirus vector sequences. Multiple silencer elements have been identified in retrovirus LTR and *gag* sequences [Challita et al., 1995; Osborne et al., 1999]. Osborne et al also demonstrate that deletions in the SIN retrovirus vectors are not enough to remove all the silencer elements [Osborne et al., 1999]. Transgene experiments show that both retrovirus and Lentivirus sequences are dominant silencers in both transgenic mice and *Drosophilia* [Pannell et al., 2000]. Direct evidence comes from blocking of retrovirus silencers by insulators. After the genomic position effect is blocked, retrovirus sequences are still silenced in transgenic mice [Yao et al., 2003]. Our and other results also show that flanking the retrovirus vector with insulators failed to avoid silencing on both retrovirus and Lentivirus vectors [Emery et al., 2000; Ramezani et al., 2003; Yannaki et al., 2002; Yao et al., 2003].

Present models account for transgene expression variegation by proposing that the cell equates the balance between positive and negative factors located in both the transgene and the flanking sequences [Dillon and Festenstein, 2002]. We propose that this can be readily applied to retrovirus silencing. The silencer elements in retrovirus vectors are dominant elements that recruit negative factors in stem cells. The transgenes harbored in the vectors bear positive elements such as enhancer, promoter or LCR sequences. The integration site flanking sequences can be either positive or negative. The final expressing state of the transgene is the sum of all the negative and positive effects of all of the recruited factors. We proposed that a negative integration environment permits the establishment of silent chromatin on the integrated retrovirus vectors. On the other hand, when a provirus locates in a constantly active domain the chromatin environment will not permit the silencing machinery to establish silent chromatin on the retrovirus vector. As a result, the integrated retrovirus will continue to express even after differentiation, but only to low levels because of continued binding by the stem cell silencing factors. The variegated retrovirus vector may reflect the recruitment of silencing proteins by retrovirus silencers into an otherwise active chromatin environment that is near heterochromatin. During differentiation of ES cells, some genomic domains are progressively silenced [Rasmussen, 2003]. Correspondingly, provirus located in these regions may also be shut down resulting in extinction (Figure 4.).

Since the Mo-MuLV enhancer is almost non-functional in ES cells [Tsukiyama et al., 1989], the balance of the positive and negative factors lean to the negative side. This explains why Mo-MuLV can induce stronger silencing compared to MSCV [Hawley, 1994]. This balance model also can explain why the inclusion of LCR or MARs elements in retrovirus vectors can limit silencing effects [Emery et al., 2002; Ma et al., 2003; Ramezani et al., 2003]. This model emphasizes the silencers as the main determinant of the retrovirus silencing, but does not underestimate the importance of the integration site flanking sequences.

7. Future Directions

7.1. Role of integration site in determining retrovirus silencing

Our model proposes that the integration site is involved to some degree in the decision to silence retrovirus in stem cells. To test this model, the relationship between retrovirus vector expression status and its integration site needs to be investigated. The effect of the integrated retrovirus vector on the flanking genomic genes also needs to be studied. The inverse PCR technique has been combined with bioinformatics research to successfully identify large number of integration sites in retrovirus and Lentivirus infected bulk cell populations [Schroder et al., 2002; Wu et al., 2003]. After identification of the integration sites and their chromatin features, the relationship between retrovirus silencing and the integration environment can be studied.

7.2. Retrovirus silencing in somatic stem cells

Because of the ethical problems associated with using human ES cells, somatic stem cells have been the center of attention for gene therapy. The finding of somatic stem cell plasticity

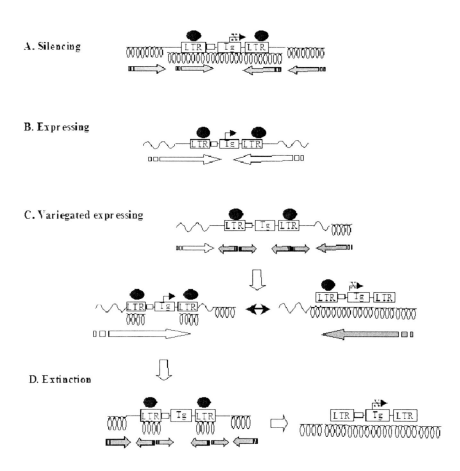

Figure 4. Retrovirus silencing hypothetical model

A). When the retrovirus vector is integrated into heterochromatin, the formation of silent chromatin on the LTRs and the spread of flanking heterochromatin establish silencing. B). When the retrovirus vector is integrated into extremely active euchromatin, the spread of active effects from the flanking gene inhibits the establishment of silent chromatin on LTRs. C). When the retrovirus vector integrates into euchromatin, variegated expression will be established by the balance of the spreading of silent effects from LTRs and the spread of active effects from euchromatin. D). During differentiation, the flanking euchromatin turns into heterochromatin and the transgene will be extinguished by the spreading of silencing effects from both LTRs and flanking heterochromatin. The black circle represents silencing factors.

[Bjornson et al., 1999; Martin-Rendon and Watt, 2003] further emphasizes the importance of somatic stem cell studies. Although retrovirus and Lentivirus silencing have been documented in HSC, the understanding of this silencing and its mechanisms are limited. The lack of identity of HSC makes it difficult to monitor single HSC clones and their differentiation. As a result, the identification of different silencing phenomena and investigation of their mechanisms are restricted. In addition, whether other somatic stem cells retain retrovirus silencing pathways that may interfere with gene therapy needs to be addressed. The neural stem cell (NSC) has the potential to be used to study retrovirus silencing. Theoretically, a single neurosphere can be derived from a single NSC. Therefore, isolation of single NSC derived neurospheres can be used to identify retrovirus silencing or variegation. NSC have the potential to differentiate into three types of neural cells: astrocytes, oligodendrocytes and neurons [McKay, 1997]. Differentiation of single NSC derived neurospheres can be used to study retrovirus extinction.

8. Final Conclusions

In conclusion, retrovirus and Lentivirus silencing are heterogeneous epigenetic phenomena that involve induction of inheritable silent chromatin on integrated retroviruses. While every integrated retrovirus has the potential to be silenced, silent chromatin only can be established in a permissive genomic environment. Retrovirus silencing is achieved by cooperation of multiple cellular gene repression mechanisms to induce either static or dynamic silent chromatin conformations resulting in retrovirus silencing and variegated expression. Silent chromatin serves as the inheritable epigenetic mark that can be passed through DNA replication during cell division. The silent chromatin formed on the retrovirus vector sequences can spread into the flanking genes. Spread of retrovirus silencing can be blocked by insulator elements. Finally, insulator elements with retrovirus silencer blocking activity can be used to design silencing resistant retrovirus and Lentivirus vectors.

References

Allen, G. C., Spiker, S., and Thompson, W. F. (2000). Use of matrix attachment regions (MARs) to minimize transgene silencing. *Plant Mol Biol 43*, 361-376.

Ayyanathan, K., Lechner, M. S., Bell, P., Maul, G. G., Schultz, D. C., Yamada, Y., Tanaka, K., Torigoe, K., and Rauscher, F. J., 3rd (2003). Regulated recruitment of HP1 to a euchromatic gene induces mitotically heritable, epigenetic gene silencing: a mammalian cell culture model of gene variegation. *Genes Dev 17*, 1855-1869.

Bacheler, L., Jaenisch, R., and Fan, H. (1979). Highly inducible cell lines derived from mice genetically transmitting the Moloney murine leukemia virus genome. *J Virol 29*, 896-906.

Ballestar, E., and Wolffe, A. P. (2001). Methyl-CpG-binding proteins. Targeting specific gene repression. *Eur J Biochem 268*, 1-6.

Barklis, E., Mulligan, R. C., and Jaenisch, R. (1986). Chromosomal position or virus mutation permits retrovirus expression in embryonal carcinoma cells. *Cell 47*, 391-399.

Barolo, S., and Levine, M. (1997). hairy mediates dominant repression in the Drosophila embryo. *Embo J 16*, 2883-2891.

Bell, A. C., and Felsenfeld, G. (1999). Stopped at the border: boundaries and insulators. Curr *Opin Genet Dev 9*, 191-198.

Bell, A. C., West, A. G., and Felsenfeld, G. (1999). The protein CTCF is required for the enhancer blocking activity of vertebrate insulators. *Cell 98*, 387-396.

Berger, S. L. (2002). Histone modifications in transcriptional regulation. *Curr Opin Genet Dev 12*, 142-148.

Bestor, T. H. (1990). DNA methylation: evolution of a bacterial immune function into a regulator of gene expression and genome structure in higher eukaryotes. *Philos Trans R Soc Lond B Biol Sci 326*, 179-187.

Bhattacharjee, R. N., Banks, G. C., Trotter, K. W., Lee, H. L., and Archer, T. K. (2001). Histone H1 phosphorylation by Cdk2 selectively modulates mouse mammary tumor virus transcription through chromatin remodeling. *Mol Cell Biol 21*, 5417-5425.

Bird, A. P., and Wolffe, A. P. (1999). Methylation-induced repression--belts, braces, and chromatin. *Cell 99*, 451-454.

Bjornson, C. R., Rietze, R. L., Reynolds, B. A., Magli, M. C., and Vescovi, A. L. (1999). Turning brain into blood: a hematopoietic fate adopted by adult neural stem cells in vivo. *Science 283*, 534-537.

Bonifer, C., Yannoutsos, N., Kruger, G., Grosveld, F., and Sippel, A. E. (1994). Dissection of the locus control function located on the chicken lysozyme gene domain in transgenic mice. *Nucleic Acids Res 22*, 4202-4210.

Breindl, M., Doehmer, J., Willecke, K., Dausman, J., and Jaenisch, R. (1979). Germ line integration of Moloney leukemia virus: identification of the chromosomal integration site. *Proc Natl Acad Sci* U S A *76*, 1938-1942.

Breindl, M., Harbers, K., and Jaenisch, R. (1984). Retrovirus-induced lethal mutation in collagen I gene of mice is associated with an altered chromatin structure. *Cell 38*, 9-16.

Breindl, M., and Jaenisch, R. (1979). Conformation of Moloney murine leukaemia proviral sequences in chromatin from leukaemic and nonleukaemic cells. *Nature 277*, 320-322.

Buchschacher, G. L., Jr., and Wong-Staal, F. (2000). Development of lentiviral vectors for gene therapy for human diseases. *Blood 95*, 2499-2504.

Burcin, M., Arnold, R., Lutz, M., Kaiser, B., Runge, D., Lottspeich, F., Filippova, G. N., Lobanenkov, V. V., and Renkawitz, R. (1997). Negative protein 1, which is required for function of the chicken lysozyme gene silencer in conjunction with hormone receptors, is identical to the multivalent zinc finger repressor CTCF. *Mol Cell Biol 17*, 1281-1288.

Byrd, K., and Corces, V. G. (2003). Visualization of chromatin domains created by the gypsy insulator of Drosophila. *J Cell Biol 162*, 565-574.

Cai, H., and Levine, M. (1995). Modulation of enhancer-promoter interactions by insulators in the Drosophila embryo. *Nature 376*, 533-536.

Cai, H. N., and Shen, P. (2001). Effects of cis arrangement of chromatin insulators on enhancer-blocking activity. *Science 291*, 493-495.

Cao, R., Wang, L., Wang, H., Xia, L., Erdjument-Bromage, H., Tempst, P., Jones, R. S., and Zhang, Y. (2002). Role of histone H3 lysine 27 methylation in Polycomb-group silencing. *Science 298*, 1039-1043.

Carlone, D. L., and Skalnik, D. G. (2001). CpG binding protein is crucial for early embryonic development. *Mol Cell Biol 21*, 7601-7606.

Challita, P. M., and Kohn, D. B. (1994). Lack of expression from a retroviral vector after transduction of murine hematopoietic stem cells is associated with methylation in vivo. *Proc Natl Acad Sci* U S A *91*, 2567-2571.

Challita, P. M., Skelton, D., el-Khoueiry, A., Yu, X. J., Weinberg, K., and Kohn, D. B. (1995). Multiple modifications in cis elements of the long terminal repeat of retroviral vectors lead to increased expression and decreased DNA methylation in embryonic carcinoma cells. *J Virol 69*, 748-755.

Chen, W. G., Chang, Q., Lin, Y., Meissner, A., West, A. E., Griffith, E. C., Jaenisch, R., and Greenberg, M. E. (2003). Derepression of BDNF transcription involves calcium-dependent phosphorylation of MeCP2. *Science 302*, 885-889.

Cherry, S. R., Biniszkiewicz, D., van Parijs, L., Baltimore, D., and Jaenisch, R. (2000). Retroviral expression in embryonic stem cells and hematopoietic stem cells. *Mol Cell Biol 20*, 7419-7426.

Cheung, P., Allis, C. D., and Sassone-Corsi, P. (2000). Signaling to chromatin through histone modifications. *Cell 103*, 263-271.

Chicurel, M. (2000). Virology. Probing HIV's elusive activities within the host cell. *Science 290*, 1876-1879.

Chung, J. H., Bell, A. C., and Felsenfeld, G. (1997). Characterization of the chicken beta-globin insulator. *Proc Natl Acad Sci* U S A *94*, 575-580.

Chung, J. H., Whiteley, M., and Felsenfeld, G. (1993). A 5' element of the chicken beta-globin domain serves as an insulator in human erythroid cells and protects against position effect in Drosophila. *Cell 74*, 505-514.

Colicelli, J., and Goff, S. P. (1986). Isolation of a recombinant murine leukemia virus utilizing a new primer tRNA. *J Virol 57*, 37-45.

Colicelli, J., and Goff, S. P. (1987). Identification of endogenous retroviral sequences as potential donors for recombinational repair of mutant retroviruses: positions of crossover points. *Virology 160*, 518-522.

Crane-Robinson, C., Myers, F. A., Hebbes, T. R., Clayton, A. L., and Thorne, A. W. (1999). Chromatin immunoprecipitation assays in acetylation mapping of higher eukaryotes. *Methods Enzymol 304*, 533-547.

Czermin, B., Melfi, R., McCabe, D., Seitz, V., Imhof, A., and Pirrotta, V. (2002). Drosophila enhancer of Zeste/ESC complexes have a histone H3 methyltransferase activity that marks chromosomal Polycomb sites. *Cell 111*, 185-196.

Dickinson, L. A., Joh, T., Kohwi, Y., and Kohwi-Shigematsu, T. (1992). A tissue-specific MAR/SAR DNA-binding protein with unusual binding site recognition. *Cell 70*, 631-645.

Dillon, N., and Festenstein, R. (2002). Unravelling heterochromatin: competition between positive and negative factors regulates accessibility. *Trends Genet 18*, 252-258.

Doerfler, W. (1991). Patterns of DNA methylation--evolutionary vestiges of foreign DNA inactivation as a host defense mechanism. A proposal. *Biol Chem Hoppe Seyler 372*, 557-564.

Dull, T., Zufferey, R., Kelly, M., Mandel, R. J., Nguyen, M., Trono, D., and Naldini, L. (1998). A third-generation lentivirus vector with a conditional packaging system. *J Virol 72*, 8463-8471.

Eissenberg, J. C., and Elgin, S. C. (2000). The HP1 protein family: getting a grip on chromatin. *Curr Opin Genet Dev 10*, 204-210.

Ellis, J., Pasceri, P., Tan-Un, K. C., Wu, X., Harper, A., Fraser, P., and Grosveld, F. (1997). Evaluation of beta-globin gene therapy constructs in single copy transgenic mice. *Nucleic Acids Res 25*, 1296-1302.

Emery, D. W., Yannaki, E., Tubb, J., Nishino, T., Li, Q., and Stamatoyannopoulos, G. (2002). Development of virus vectors for gene therapy of beta chain hemoglobinopathies: flanking with a chromatin insulator reduces gamma-globin gene silencing in vivo. *Blood 100*, 2012-2019.

Emery, D. W., Yannaki, E., Tubb, J., and Stamatoyannopoulos, G. (2000). A chromatin insulator protects retrovirus vectors from chromosomal position effects. *Proc Natl Acad Sci* U S A *97*, 9150-9155.

Festenstein, R., Sharghi-Namini, S., Fox, M., Roderick, K., Tolaini, M., Norton, T., Saveliev, A., Kioussis, D., and Singh, P. (1999). Heterochromatin protein 1 modifies mammalian PEV in a dose- and chromosomal-context-dependent manner. *Nat Genet 23*, 457-461.

Festenstein, R., Tolaini, M., Corbella, P., Mamalaki, C., Parrington, J., Fox, M., Miliou, A., Jones, M., and Kioussis, D. (1996). Locus control region function and heterochromatin-induced position effect variegation. *Science 271*, 1123-1125.

Flanagan, J. R., Becker, K. G., Ennist, D. L., Gleason, S. L., Driggers, P. H., Levi, B. Z., Appella, E., and Ozato, K. (1992). Cloning of a negative transcription factor that binds to the upstream conserved region of Moloney murine leukemia virus. *Mol Cell Biol 12*, 38-44.

Flanagan, J. R., Krieg, A. M., Max, E. E., and Khan, A. S. (1989). Negative control region at the 5' end of murine leukemia virus long terminal repeats. *Mol Cell Biol 9*, 739-746.

Fuks, F., Hurd, P. J., Deplus, R., and Kouzarides, T. (2003a). The DNA methyltransferases associate with HP1 and the SUV39H1 histone methyltransferase. *Nucleic Acids Res 31*, 2305-2312.

Fuks, F., Hurd, P. J., Wolf, D., Nan, X., Bird, A. P., and Kouzarides, T. (2003b). The methyl-CpG-binding protein MeCP2 links DNA methylation to histone methylation. *J Biol Chem 278*, 4035-4040.

Gao, G., Guo, X., and Goff, S. P. (2002). Inhibition of retroviral RNA production by ZAP, a CCCH-type zinc finger protein. *Science 297*, 1703-1706.

Gaszner, M., Vazquez, J., and Schedl, P. (1999). The Zw5 protein, a component of the scs chromatin domain boundary, is able to block enhancer-promoter interaction. *Genes Dev 13*, 2098-2107.

Gause, M., Morcillo, P., and Dorsett, D. (2001). Insulation of enhancer-promoter communication by a gypsy transposon insert in the Drosophila cut gene: cooperation between suppressor of hairy-wing and modifier of mdg4 proteins. *Mol Cell Biol 21*, 4807-4817.

Gautsch, J. W. (1980). Embryonal carcinoma stem cells lack a function required for virus replication. *Nature 285*, 110-112.

Gautsch, J. W., and Wilson, M. C. (1983). Delayed de novo methylation in teratocarcinoma suggests additional tissue-specific mechanisms for controlling gene expression. *Nature 301*, 32-37.

Gdula, D. A., Gerasimova, T. I., and Corces, V. G. (1996). Genetic and molecular analysis of the gypsy chromatin insulator of Drosophila. *Proc Natl Acad Sci* U S A *93*, 9378-9383.

Georgel, P. T., Horowitz-Scherer, R. A., Adkins, N., Woodcock, C. L., Wade, P. A., and Hansen, J. C. (2003). Chromatin compaction by human MeCP2. Assembly of novel secondary chromatin structures in the absence of DNA methylation. *J Biol Chem 278*, 32181-32188.

Gerasimova, T. I., Byrd, K., and Corces, V. G. (2000). A chromatin insulator determines the nuclear localization of DNA. *Mol Cell 6*, 1025-1035.

Geyer, P. K., and Corces, V. G. (1992). DNA position-specific repression of transcription by a Drosophila zinc finger protein. *Genes Dev 6*, 1865-1873.

Ghosh, D., Gerasimova, T. I., and Corces, V. G. (2001). Interactions between the Su(Hw) and Mod(mdg4) proteins required for gypsy insulator function. *Embo J 20*, 2518-2527.

Graziano, V., Gerchman, S. E., Schneider, D. K., and Ramakrishnan, V. (1994). Histone H1 is located in the interior of the chromatin 30-nm filament. *Nature 368*, 351-354.

Grewal, S. I., and Moazed, D. (2003). Heterochromatin and epigenetic control of gene expression. *Science 301*, 798-802.

Grez, M., Akgun, E., Hilberg, F., and Ostertag, W. (1990). Embryonic stem cell virus, a recombinant murine retrovirus with expression in embryonic stem cells. *Proc Natl Acad Sci* U S A *87*, 9202-9206.

Guenechea, G., Gan, O. I., Dorrell, C., and Dick, J. E. (2001). Distinct classes of human stem cells that differ in proliferative and self-renewal potential. *Nat Immunol 2*, 75-82.

Hamaguchi, I., Woods, N. B., Panagopoulos, I., Andersson, E., Mikkola, H., Fahlman, C., Zufferey, R., Carlsson, L., Trono, D., and Karlsson, S. (2000). Lentivirus vector gene expression during ES cell-derived hematopoietic development in vitro. *J Virol 74*, 10778-10784.

Hart, C. M., Zhao, K., and Laemmli, U. K. (1997). The scs' boundary element: characterization of boundary element-associated factors. *Mol Cell Biol 17*, 999-1009.

Hata, K., Okano, M., Lei, H., and Li, E. (2002). Dnmt3L cooperates with the Dnmt3 family of de novo DNA methyltransferases to establish maternal imprints in mice. *Development 129*, 1983-1993.

Hawley, R. G. (1994). High-titer retroviral vectors for efficient transduction of functional genes into murine hematopoietic stem cells. *Ann N Y Acad Sci 716*, 327-330.

Hilberg, F., Stocking, C., Ostertag, W., and Grez, M. (1987). Functional analysis of a retroviral host-range mutant: altered long terminal repeat sequences allow expression in embryonal carcinoma cells. *Proc Natl Acad Sci* U S A *84*, 5232-5236.

Horn, P. J., Carruthers, L. M., Logie, C., Hill, D. A., Solomon, M. J., Wade, P. A., Imbalzano, A. N., Hansen, J. C., and Peterson, C. L. (2002). Phosphorylation of linker histones regulates ATP-dependent chromatin remodeling enzymes. *Nat Struct Biol 9*, 263-267.

Hung, M. S., Karthikeyan, N., Huang, B., Koo, H. C., Kiger, J., and Shen, C. J. (1999). Drosophila proteins related to vertebrate DNA (5-cytosine) methyltransferases. *Proc Natl Acad Sci* U S A *96*, 11940-11945.

Iida, T., Suetake, I., Tajima, S., Morioka, H., Ohta, S., Obuse, C., and Tsurimoto, T. (2002). PCNA clamp facilitates action of DNA cytosine methyltransferase 1 on hemimethylated DNA. *Genes Cells 7*, 997-1007.

Illmensee, K., and Mintz, B. (1976). Totipotency and normal differentiation of single teratocarcinoma cells cloned by injection into blastocysts. *Proc Natl Acad Sci* U S A *73*, 549-553.

Iwakuma, T., Cui, Y., and Chang, L. J. (1999). Self-inactivating lentiviral vectors with U3 and U5 modifications. *Virology 261*, 120-132.

Jackson, J. P., Lindroth, A. M., Cao, X., and Jacobsen, S. E. (2002). Control of CpNpG DNA methylation by the KRYPTONITE histone H3 methyltransferase. *Nature 416*, 556-560.

Jaenisch, R. (1980). Retroviruses and embryogenesis: microinjection of Moloney leukemia virus into midgestation mouse embryos. *Cell 19*, 181-188.

Jaenisch, R., Fan, H., and Croker, B. (1975). Infection of preimplantation mouse embryos and of newborn mice with leukemia virus: tissue distribution of viral DNA and RNA and leukemogenesis in the adult animal. *Proc Natl Acad Sci* U S A *72*, 4008-4012.

Jahner, D., Stuhlmann, H., Stewart, C. L., Harbers, K., Lohler, J., Simon, I., and Jaenisch, R. (1982). De novo methylation and expression of retroviral genomes during mouse embryogenesis. *Nature 298*, 623-628.

Jones, P. L., Veenstra, G. J., Wade, P. A., Vermaak, D., Kass, S. U., Landsberger, N., Strouboulis, J., and Wolffe, A. P. (1998). Methylated DNA and MeCP2 recruit histone deacetylase to repress transcription. *Nat Genet 19*, 187-191.

Karymov, M. A., Tomschik, M., Leuba, S. H., Caiafa, P., and Zlatanova, J. (2001). DNA methylation-dependent chromatin fiber compaction in vivo and in vitro: requirement for linker histone. *Faseb J 15*, 2631-2641.

Kellum, R., and Schedl, P. (1991). A position-effect assay for boundaries of higher order chromosomal domains. *Cell 64*, 941-950.

Kellum, R., and Schedl, P. (1992). A group of scs elements function as domain boundaries in an enhancer-blocking assay. *Mol Cell Biol 12*, 2424-2431.

Kim, V. N., Mitrophanous, K., Kingsman, S. M., and Kingsman, A. J. (1998). Minimal requirement for a lentivirus vector based on human immunodeficiency virus type 1. *J Virol 72*, 811-816.

Kioussis, D., and Festenstein, R. (1997). Locus control regions: overcoming heterochromatin-induced gene inactivation in mammals. *Curr Opin Genet Dev 7*, 614-619.

Klenova, E. M., Fagerlie, S., Filippova, G. N., Kretzner, L., Goodwin, G. H., Loring, G., Neiman, P. E., and Lobanenkov, V. V. (1998). Characterization of the chicken CTCF genomic locus, and initial study of the cell cycle-regulated promoter of the gene. *J Biol Chem 273*, 26571-26579.

Klug, C. A., Cheshier, S., and Weissman, I. L. (2000). Inactivation of a GFP retrovirus occurs at multiple levels in long-term repopulating stem cells and their differentiated progeny. *Blood 96*, 894-901.

Laker, C., Meyer, J., Schopen, A., Friel, J., Heberlein, C., Ostertag, W., and Stocking, C. (1998). Host cis-mediated extinction of a retrovirus permissive for expression in embryonal stem cells during differentiation. *J Virol 72*, 339-348.

Lange, C., and Blankenstein, T. (1997). Loss of retroviral gene expression in bone marrow reconstituted mice correlates with down-regulation of gene expression in long-term culture initiating cells. *Gene Ther 4*, 303-308.

Leonhardt, H., Page, A. W., Weier, H. U., and Bestor, T. H. (1992). A targeting sequence directs DNA methyltransferase to sites of DNA replication in mammalian nuclei. *Cell 71*, 865-873.

Lever, M. A., Th'ng, J. P., Sun, X., and Hendzel, M. J. (2000). Rapid exchange of histone H1.1 on chromatin in living human cells. *Nature 408*, 873-876.

Lewis, J. D., Meehan, R. R., Henzel, W. J., Maurer-Fogy, I., Jeppesen, P., Klein, F., and Bird, A. (1992). Purification, sequence, and cellular localization of a novel chromosomal protein that binds to methylated DNA. *Cell 69*, 905-914.

Li, E., Bestor, T. H., and Jaenisch, R. (1992). Targeted mutation of the DNA methyltransferase gene results in embryonic lethality. *Cell 69*, 915-926.

Liang, G., Chan, M. F., Tomigahara, Y., Tsai, Y. C., Gonzales, F. A., Li, E., Laird, P. W., and Jones, P. A. (2002). Cooperativity between DNA methyltransferases in the maintenance methylation of repetitive elements. *Mol Cell Biol 22*, 480-491.

Litt, M. D., Simpson, M., Gaszner, M., Allis, C. D., and Felsenfeld, G. (2001a). Correlation between histone lysine methylation and developmental changes at the chicken beta-globin locus. *Science 293*, 2453-2455.

Litt, M. D., Simpson, M., Recillas-Targa, F., Prioleau, M. N., and Felsenfeld, G. (2001b). Transitions in histone acetylation reveal boundaries of three separately regulated neighboring loci. *Embo J 20*, 2224-2235.

Liu, K., Wang, Y. F., Cantemir, C., and Muller, M. T. (2003). Endogenous assays of DNA methyltransferases: Evidence for differential activities of DNMT1, DNMT2, and DNMT3 in mammalian cells in vivo. *Mol Cell Biol 23*, 2709-2719.

Lois, C., Hong, E. J., Pease, S., Brown, E. J., and Baltimore, D. (2002). Germline transmission and tissue-specific expression of transgenes delivered by lentiviral vectors. *Science 295*, 868-872.

Lorincz, M. C., Schubeler, D., Goeke, S. C., Walters, M., Groudine, M., and Martin, D. I. (2000). Dynamic analysis of proviral induction and De Novo methylation: implications for a histone deacetylase-independent, methylation density-dependent mechanism of transcriptional repression. *Mol Cell Biol 20*, 842-850.

Lorincz, M. C., Schubeler, D., and Groudine, M. (2001). Methylation-mediated proviral silencing is associated with MeCP2 recruitment and localized histone H3 deacetylation. *Mol Cell Biol 21*, 7913-7922.

Lorincz, M. C., Schubeler, D., Hutchinson, S. R., Dickerson, D. R., and Groudine, M. (2002). DNA methylation density influences the stability of an epigenetic imprint and Dnmt3a/b-independent de novo methylation. *Mol Cell Biol 22*, 7572-7580.

Lu, L., and Tower, J. (1997). A transcriptional insulator element, the su(Hw) binding site, protects a chromosomal DNA replication origin from position effects. *Mol Cell Biol 17*, 2202-2206.

Lundgren, M., Chow, C. M., Sabbattini, P., Georgiou, A., Minaee, S., and Dillon, N. (2000). Transcription factor dosage affects changes in higher order chromatin structure associated with activation of a heterochromatic gene. *Cell 103*, 733-743.

Lutz, M., Burke, L. J., Barreto, G., Goeman, F., Greb, H., Arnold, R., Schultheiss, H., Brehm, A., Kouzarides, T., Lobanenkov, V., and Renkawitz, R. (2000). Transcriptional repression by the insulator protein CTCF involves histone deacetylases. *Nucleic Acids Res 28*, 1707-1713.

Lyko, F., Ramsahoye, B. H., and Jaenisch, R. (2000). DNA methylation in Drosophila melanogaster. *Nature 408*, 538-540.

Ma, Y., Ramezani, A., Lewis, R., Hawley, R. G., and Thomson, J. A. (2003). High-level sustained transgene expression in human embryonic stem cells using lentiviral vectors. *Stem Cells 21*, 111-117.

Mallin, D. R., Myung, J. S., Patton, J. S., and Geyer, P. K. (1998). Polycomb group repression is blocked by the Drosophila suppressor of Hairy-wing [su(Hw)] insulator. *Genetics 148*, 331-339.

Martinowich, K., Hattori, D., Wu, H., Fouse, S., He, F., Hu, Y., Fan, G., and Sun, Y. E. (2003). DNA methylation-related chromatin remodeling in activity-dependent BDNF gene regulation. *Science 302*, 890-893.

Martin-Rendon, E., and Watt, S. M. (2003). Exploitation of stem cell plasticity. *Transfus Med 13*, 325-349.

May, C., Rivella, S., Callegari, J., Heller, G., Gaensler, K. M., Luzzatto, L., and Sadelain, M. (2000). Therapeutic haemoglobin synthesis in beta-thalassaemic mice expressing lentivirus-encoded human beta-globin. *Nature 406*, 82-86.

McCune, S. L., and Townes, T. M. (1994). Retroviral vector sequences inhibit human beta-globin gene expression in transgenic mice. Nucleic Acids Res *22*, 4477-4481.

McInerney, J. M., Nawrocki, J. R., and Lowrey, C. H. (2000). Long-term silencing of retroviral vectors is resistant to reversal by trichostatin A and 5-azacytidine. *Gene Ther 7*, 653-663.

McKay, R. (1997). Stem cells in the central nervous system. *Science 276*, 66-71.

McMorrow, T., van den Wijngaard, A., Wollenschlaeger, A., van de Corput, M., Monkhorst, K., Trimborn, T., Fraser, P., van Lohuizen, M., Jenuwein, T., Djabali, M., *et al.* (2000). Activation of the beta globin locus by transcription factors and chromatin modifiers. Embo J *19*, 4986-4996.

McNairn, A. J., and Gilbert, D. M. (2003). Epigenomic replication: linking epigenetics to DNA replication. *Bioessays 25*, 647-656.

Melnikova, L., Gause, M., and Georgiev, P. (2002). The gypsy insulators flanking yellow enhancers do not form a separate transcriptional domain in Drosophila melanogaster: the enhancers can activate an isolated yellow promoter. *Genetics 160*, 1549-1560.

Mikkola, H., Woods, N. B., Sjogren, M., Helgadottir, H., Hamaguchi, I., Jacobsen, S. E., Trono, D., and Karlsson, S. (2000). Lentivirus gene transfer in murine hematopoietic progenitor cells is compromised by a delay in proviral integration and results in transduction mosaicism and heterogeneous gene expression in progeny cells. *J Virol 74*, 11911-11918.

Milne, T. A., Briggs, S. D., Brock, H. W., Martin, M. E., Gibbs, D., Allis, C. D., and Hess, J. L. (2002). MLL targets SET domain methyltransferase activity to Hox gene promoters. *Mol Cell 10*, 1107-1117.

Milot, E., Strouboulis, J., Trimborn, T., Wijgerde, M., de Boer, E., Langeveld, A., Tan-Un, K., Vergeer, W., Yannoutsos, N., Grosveld, F., and Fraser, P. (1996). Heterochromatin effects on the frequency and duration of LCR-mediated gene transcription. *Cell 87*, 105-114.

Milutinovic, S., Zhuang, Q., Niveleau, A., and Szyf, M. (2003). Epigenomic stress response. Knockdown of DNA methyltransferase 1 triggers an intra-S-phase arrest of DNA replication and induction of stress response genes. *J Biol Chem 278*, 14985-14995.

Misteli, T., Gunjan, A., Hock, R., Bustin, M., and Brown, D. T. (2000). Dynamic binding of histone H1 to chromatin in living cells. *Nature 408*, 877-881.

Miyoshi, H., Blomer, U., Takahashi, M., Gage, F. H., and Verma, I. M. (1998). Development of a self-inactivating lentivirus vector. *J Virol 72*, 8150-8157.

Moazed, D. (2001). Common themes in mechanisms of gene silencing. *Mol Cell 8*, 489-498.

Muravyova, E., Golovnin, A., Gracheva, E., Parshikov, A., Belenkaya, T., Pirrotta, V., and Georgiev, P. (2001). Loss of insulator activity by paired Su(Hw) chromatin insulators. *Science 291*, 495-498.

Mutskov, V. J., Farrell, C. M., Wade, P. A., Wolffe, A. P., and Felsenfeld, G. (2002). The barrier function of an insulator couples high histone acetylation levels with specific protection of promoter DNA from methylation. *Genes Dev 16*, 1540-1554.

Nabirochkin, S., Ossokina, M., and Heidmann, T. (1998). A nuclear matrix/scaffold attachment region co-localizes with the gypsy retrotransposon insulator sequence. *J Biol Chem 273*, 2473-2479.

Naldini, L., Blomer, U., Gallay, P., Ory, D., Mulligan, R., Gage, F. H., Verma, I. M., and Trono, D. (1996). In vivo gene delivery and stable transduction of nondividing cells by a lentiviral vector. *Science 272*, 263-267.

Naldini, L., and Verma, I. M. (2000). Lentiviral vectors. *Adv Virus Res 55*, 599-609.

Nan, X., Campoy, F. J., and Bird, A. (1997). MeCP2 is a transcriptional repressor with abundant binding sites in genomic chromatin. *Cell 88*, 471-481.

Nan, X., Meehan, R. R., and Bird, A. (1993). Dissection of the methyl-CpG binding domain from the chromosomal protein MeCP2. *Nucleic Acids Res 21*, 4886-4892.

Nan, X., Ng, H. H., Johnson, C. A., Laherty, C. D., Turner, B. M., Eisenman, R. N., and Bird, A. (1998). Transcriptional repression by the methyl-CpG-binding protein MeCP2 involves a histone deacetylase complex. *Nature 393*, 386-389.

Narlikar, G. J., Fan, H. Y., and Kingston, R. E. (2002). Cooperation between complexes that regulate chromatin structure and transcription. *Cell 108*, 475-487.

Ncr, S. S., and Travers, A. A. (1994). HMG-D, the Drosophila melanogaster homologue of HMG 1 protein, is associated with early embryonic chromatin in the absence of histone H1. *Embo J 13*, 1817-1822.

Nielsen, S. J., Schneider, R., Bauer, U. M., Bannister, A. J., Morrison, A., O'Carroll, D., Firestein, R., Cleary, M., Jenuwein, T., Herrera, R. E., and Kouzarides, T. (2001). Rb targets histone H3 methylation and HP1 to promoters. *Nature 412*, 561-565.

Niwa, O., Yokota, Y., Ishida, H., and Sugahara, T. (1983). Independent mechanisms involved in suppression of the Moloney leukemia virus genome during differentiation of murine teratocarcinoma cells. *Cell 32*, 1105-1113.

Okano, M., Bell, D. W., Haber, D. A., and Li, E. (1999). DNA methyltransferases Dnmt3a and Dnmt3b are essential for de novo methylation and mammalian development. *Cell 99*, 247-257.

Okano, M., Xie, S., and Li, E. (1998). Dnmt2 is not required for de novo and maintenance methylation of viral DNA in embryonic stem cells. *Nucleic Acids Res 26*, 2536-2540.

Osborne, C. S., Pasceri, P., Singal, R., Sukonnik, T., Ginder, G. D., and Ellis, J. (1999). Amelioration of retroviral vector silencing in locus control region beta-globin-transgenic mice and transduced F9 embryonic cells. *J Virol 73*, 5490-5496.

Pannell, D., Osborne, C. S., Yao, S., Sukonnik, T., Pasceri, P., Karaiskakis, A., Okano, M., Li, E., Lipshitz, H. D., and Ellis, J. (2000). Retrovirus vector silencing is de novo methylase independent and marked by a repressive histone code. *Embo J 19*, 5884-5894.

Pasceri, P., Pannell, D., Wu, X., and Ellis, J. (1998). Full activity from human beta-globin locus control region transgenes requires 5'HS1, distal beta-globin promoter, and 3' beta-globin sequences. *Blood 92*, 653-663.

Peries, J., Debons-Guillemin, M. C., Canivet, M., Emanoil-Ravicovitch, R., Tavitian, A., and Boiron, M. (1977). [Multiplication of murine C-type viruses in mouse teratocarcinoma cell lines]. *Nouv Rev Fr Hematol Blood Cells 18*, 383-390.

Peters, A. H., O'Carroll, D., Scherthan, H., Mechtler, K., Sauer, S., Schofer, C., Weipoltshammer, K., Pagani, M., Lachner, M., Kohlmaier, A., *et al.* (2001). Loss of the Suv39h histone methyltransferases impairs mammalian heterochromatin and genome stability. *Cell 107*, 323-337.

Petersen, R., Kempler, G., and Barklis, E. (1991). A stem cell-specific silencer in the primer-binding site of a retrovirus. *Mol Cell Biol 11*, 1214-1221.

Pfeifer, A., Ikawa, M., Dayn, Y., and Verma, I. M. (2002). Transgenesis by lentiviral vectors: lack of gene silencing in mammalian embryonic stem cells and preimplantation embryos. *Proc Natl Acad Sci* U S A *99*, 2140-2145.

Pirrotta, V. (1998). Polycombing the genome: PcG, trxG, and chromatin silencing. *Cell 93*, 333-336.

Prioleau, M. N., Nony, P., Simpson, M., and Felsenfeld, G. (1999). An insulator element and condensed chromatin region separate the chicken beta-globin locus from an independently regulated erythroid-specific folate receptor gene. *Embo J 18*, 4035-4048.

Quinonez, R., and Sutton, R. E. (2002). Lentiviral vectors for gene delivery into cells. *DNA Cell Biol 21*, 937-951.

Ramezani, A., and Hawley, R. G. (2003). Human immunodeficiency virus type 1-based vectors for gene delivery to human hematopoietic stem cells. *Methods Mol Med 76*, 467-492.

Ramezani, A., Hawley, T. S., and Hawley, R. G. (2003). Performance- and safety-enhanced lentiviral vectors containing the human interferon-beta scaffold attachment region and the chicken beta-globin insulator. *Blood 101*, 4717-4724.

Rasmussen, T. P. (2003). Embryonic stem cell differentiation: A chromatin perspective. *Reprod Biol Endocrinol 1*, 100.

Rea, S., Eisenhaber, F., O'Carroll, D., Strahl, B. D., Sun, Z. W., Schmid, M., Opravil, S., Mechtler, K., Ponting, C. P., Allis, C. D., and Jenuwein, T. (2000). Regulation of chromatin structure by site-specific histone H3 methyltransferases. *Nature 406*, 593-599.

Recillas-Targa, F., Pikaart, M. J., Burgess-Beusse, B., Bell, A. C., Litt, M. D., West, A. G., Gaszner, M., and Felsenfeld, G. (2002). Position-effect protection and enhancer blocking by the chicken beta-globin insulator are separable activities. *Proc Natl Acad Sci* U S A *99*, 6883-6888.

Reid, J. L., Iyer, V. R., Brown, P. O., and Struhl, K. (2000). Coordinate regulation of yeast ribosomal protein genes is associated with targeted recruitment of Esa1 histone acetylase. *Mol Cell 6*, 1297-1307.

Rivella, S., Callegari, J. A., May, C., Tan, C. W., and Sadelain, M. (2000). The cHS4 insulator increases the probability of retroviral expression at random chromosomal integration sites. *J Virol 74*, 4679-4687.

Robbins, P. B., Skelton, D. C., Yu, X. J., Halene, S., Leonard, E. H., and Kohn, D. B. (1998). Consistent, persistent expression from modified retroviral vectors in murine hematopoietic stem cells. *Proc Natl Acad Sci* U S A *95*, 10182-10187.

Roth, S. Y., Denu, J. M., and Allis, C. D. (2001). Histone acetyltransferases. *Annu Rev Biochem 70*, 81-120.

Russo, V. E. A., Martienssen, R.A. and Riggs, A.D. (1996). Epigenetic Mechanisms of Gene Regulation. In *Cold Spring Harbor Laboratory Press*, pp. 1-5.

Santos, F., Hendrich, B., Reik, W., and Dean, W. (2002). Dynamic reprogramming of DNA methylation in the early mouse embryo. *Dev Biol 241*, 172-182.

Schilz, A. J., Brouns, G., Knoss, H., Ottmann, O. G., Hoelzer, D., Fauser, A. A., Thrasher, A. J., and Grez, M. (1998). High efficiency gene transfer to human hematopoietic SCID-repopulating cells under serum-free conditions. *Blood 92*, 3163-3171.

Schotta, G., Ebert, A., Krauss, V., Fischer, A., Hoffmann, J., Rea, S., Jenuwein, T., Dorn, R., and Reuter, G. (2002). Central role of Drosophila SU(VAR)3-9 in histone H3-K9 methylation and heterochromatic gene silencing. *Embo J 21*, 1121-1131.

Schramke, V., and Allshire, R. (2003). Hairpin RNAs and retrotransposon LTRs effect RNAi and chromatin-based gene silencing. *Science 301*, 1069-1074.

Schroder, A. R., Shinn, P., Chen, H., Berry, C., Ecker, J. R., and Bushman, F. (2002). HIV-1 integration in the human genome favors active genes and local hotspots. *Cell 110*, 521-529.

Sewalt, R. G., Lachner, M., Vargas, M., Hamer, K. M., den Blaauwen, J. L., Hendrix, T., Melcher, M., Schweizer, D., Jenuwein, T., and Otte, A. P. (2002). Selective interactions between vertebrate polycomb homologs and the SUV39H1 histone lysine methyltransferase suggest that histone H3-K9 methylation contributes to chromosomal targeting of Polycomb group proteins. *Mol Cell Biol 22*, 5539-5553.

Shen, X., and Gorovsky, M. A. (1996). Linker histone H1 regulates specific gene expression but not global transcription in vivo. *Cell 86*, 475-483.

Shore, D. (2000). The Sir2 protein family: A novel deacetylase for gene silencing and more. *Proc Natl Acad Sci* U S A *97*, 14030-14032.

Simon, D., Stuhlmann, H., Jahner, D., Wagner, H., Werner, E., and Jaenisch, R. (1983). Retrovirus genomes methylated by mammalian but not bacterial methylase are non-infectious. *Nature 304*, 275-277.

Sirven, A., Pflumio, F., Zennou, V., Titeux, M., Vainchenker, W., Coulombel, L., Dubart-Kupperschmitt, A., and Charneau, P. (2000). The human immunodeficiency virus type-1 central DNA flap is a crucial determinant for lentiviral vector nuclear import and gene transduction of human hematopoietic stem cells. *Blood 96*, 4103-4110.

Sirven, A., Ravet, E., Charneau, P., Zennou, V., Coulombel, L., Guetard, D., Pflumio, F., and Dubart-Kupperschmitt, A. (2001). Enhanced transgene expression in cord blood CD34(+)-derived hematopoietic cells, including developing T cells and NOD/SCID mouse repopulating cells, following transduction with modified trip lentiviral vectors. *Mol Ther 3*, 438-448.

Speck, N. A., and Baltimore, D. (1987). Six distinct nuclear factors interact with the 75-base-pair repeat of the Moloney murine leukemia virus enhancer. *Mol Cell Biol 7*, 1101-1110.

Speers, W. C., Gautsch, J. W., and Dixon, F. J. (1980). Silent infection of murine embryonal carcinoma cells by Moloney murine leukemia virus. *Virology 105*, 241-244.

Stancheva, I., Collins, A. L., Van den Veyver, I. B., Zoghbi, H., and Meehan, R. R. (2003). A mutant form of MeCP2 protein associated with human Rett syndrome cannot be displaced from methylated DNA by notch in Xenopus embryos. *Mol Cell 12*, 425-435.

Stewart, C. L., Stuhlmann, H., Jahner, D., and Jaenisch, R. (1982). De novo methylation, expression, and infectivity of retroviral genomes introduced into embryonal carcinoma cells. *Proc Natl Acad Sci* U S A *79*, 4098-4102.

Strahl, B. D., and Allis, C. D. (2000). The language of covalent histone modifications. *Nature 403*, 41-45.

Swindle, C. S., Kim, H. G., and Klug, C. A. (2004). Mutation of CpGs in the Murine Stem Cell Virus Retroviral Vector Long Terminal Repeat Represses Silencing in Embryonic Stem Cells. *J Biol Chem 279*, 34-41.

Tachibana, M., Sugimoto, K., Fukushima, T., and Shinkai, Y. (2001). Set domain-containing protein, G9a, is a novel lysine-preferring mammalian histone methyltransferase with hyperactivity and specific selectivity to lysines 9 and 27 of histone H3. *J Biol Chem 276*, 25309-25317.

Teich, N. M., Weiss, R. A., Martin, G. R., and Lowy, D. R. (1977). Virus infection of murine teratocarcinoma stem cell lines. *Cell 12*, 973-982.

Trevisan, M., and Iscove, N. N. (1995). Phenotypic analysis of murine long-term hemopoietic reconstituting cells quantitated competitively in vivo and comparison with more advanced colony-forming progeny. *J Exp Med 181*, 93-103.

Tsukiyama, T., and Niwa, O. (1992). Isolation of high affinity cellular targets of the embryonal LTR binding protein, an undifferentiated embryonal carcinoma cell-specific repressor of Moloney leukemia virus. *Nucleic Acids Res 20*, 1477-1482.

Tsukiyama, T., Niwa, O., and Yokoro, K. (1989). Mechanism of suppression of the long terminal repeat of Moloney leukemia virus in mouse embryonal carcinoma cells. *Mol Cell Biol 9*, 4670-4676.

Uchida, N., Sutton, R. E., Friera, A. M., He, D., Reitsma, M. J., Chang, W. C., Veres, G., Scollay, R., and Weissman, I. L. (1998). HIV, but not murine leukemia virus, vectors mediate high efficiency gene transfer into freshly isolated G0/G1 human hematopoietic stem cells. *Proc Natl Acad Sci* U S A *95*, 11939-11944.

Udvardy, A., Maine, E., and Schedl, P. (1985). The 87A7 chromomere. Identification of novel chromatin structures flanking the heat shock locus that may define the boundaries of higher order domains. *J Mol Biol 185*, 341-358.

Urieli-Shoval, S., Gruenbaum, Y., Sedat, J., and Razin, A. (1982). The absence of detectable methylated bases in Drosophila melanogaster DNA. *FEBS Lett 146*, 148-152.

van der Vlag, J., den Blaauwen, J. L., Sewalt, R. G., van Driel, R., and Otte, A. P. (2000). Transcriptional repression mediated by polycomb group proteins and other chromatin-associated repressors is selectively blocked by insulators. *J Biol Chem 275*, 697-704.

Verma, I. M., and Somia, N. (1997). Gene therapy -- promises, problems and prospects. *Nature 389*, 239-242.

Vogelauer, M., Wu, J., Suka, N., and Grunstein, M. (2000). Global histone acetylation and deacetylation in yeast. Nature *408*, 495-498.

Voo, K. S., Carlone, D. L., Jacobsen, B. M., Flodin, A., and Skalnik, D. G. (2000). Cloning of a mammalian transcriptional activator that binds unmethylated CpG motifs and shares a CXXC domain with DNA methyltransferase, human trithorax, and methyl-CpG binding domain protein 1. *Mol Cell Biol 20*, 2108-2121.

Walsh, C. P., and Bestor, T. H. (1999). Cytosine methylation and mammalian development. *Genes Dev 13*, 26-34.

Walsh, C. P., Chaillet, J. R., and Bestor, T. H. (1998). Transcription of IAP endogenous retroviruses is constrained by cytosine methylation. *Nat Genet 20*, 116-117.

Weintraub, H., and Groudine, M. (1976). Chromosomal subunits in active genes have an altered conformation. *Science 193*, 848-856.

Wolffe, A. P., and Guschin, D. (2000). Review: chromatin structural features and targets that regulate transcription. *J Struct Biol 129*, 102-122.

Wolffe, A. P., and Matzke, M. A. (1999). Epigenetics: regulation through repression. *Science 286*, 481-486.

Woods, N. B., Fahlman, C., Mikkola, H., Hamaguchi, I., Olsson, K., Zufferey, R., Jacobsen, S. E., Trono, D., and Karlsson, S. (2000). Lentiviral gene transfer into primary and secondary NOD/SCID repopulating cells. *Blood 96*, 3725-3733.

Wu, X., Li, Y., Crise, B., and Burgess, S. M. (2003). Transcription start regions in the human genome are favored targets for MLV integration. *Science 300*, 1749-1751.

Xie, S., Wang, Z., Okano, M., Nogami, M., Li, Y., He, W. W., Okumura, K., and Li, E. (1999). Cloning, expression and chromosome locations of the human DNMT3 gene family. *Gene 236*, 87-95.

Yannaki, E., Tubb, J., Aker, M., Stamatoyannopoulos, G., and Emery, D. W. (2002). Topological constraints governing the use of the chicken HS4 chromatin insulator in oncoretrovirus vectors. *Mol Ther 5*, 589-598.

Yao, S., Osborne, C. S., Bharadwaj, R. R., Pasceri, P., Sukonnik, T., Pannell, D., Recillas-Targa, F., West, A. G., and Ellis, J. (2003). Retrovirus silencer blocking by the cHS4 insulator is CTCF independent. *Nucleic Acids Res 31*, 5317-5323.

Yao, S., Sukonnik, T., Kean, T., Bharadwaj R.R., Pasceri P. and Ellis J. (2004). Retrovirus silencing, variegation, extinction and memory are controlled by dynamic interplay of multiple epigenetic modifications. *Mol Ther* In Press.

Yoder, J. A., Soman, N. S., Verdine, G. L., and Bestor, T. H. (1997a). DNA (cytosine-5)-methyltransferases in mouse cells and tissues. Studies with a mechanism-based probe. *J Mol Biol 270*, 385-395.

Yoder, J. A., Walsh, C. P., and Bestor, T. H. (1997b). Cytosine methylation and the ecology of intragenomic parasites. *Trends Genet 13*, 335-340.

Yu, S. F., von Ruden, T., Kantoff, P. W., Garber, C., Seiberg, M., Ruther, U., Anderson, W. F., Wagner, E. F., and Gilboa, E. (1986). Self-inactivating retroviral vectors designed for transfer of whole genes into mammalian cells. *Proc Natl Acad Sci* U S A *83*, 3194-3198.

Zentilin, L., Qin, G., Tafuro, S., Dinauer, M. C., Baum, C., and Giacca, M. (2000). Variegation of retroviral vector gene expression in myeloid cells. *Gene Ther 7*, 153-166.

Zhao, K., Hart, C. M., and Laemmli, U. K. (1995). Visualization of chromosomal domains with boundary element-associated factor BEAF-32. *Cell 81*, 879-889.

Zufferey, R., Donello, J. E., Trono, D., and Hope, T. J. (1999). Woodchuck hepatitis virus posttranscriptional regulatory element enhances expression of transgenes delivered by retroviral vectors. *J Virol 73*, 2886-2892.

Zufferey, R., Dull, T., Mandel, R. J., Bukovsky, A., Quiroz, D., Naldini, L., and Trono, D. (1998). Self-inactivating lentivirus vector for safe and efficient in vivo gene delivery. *J Virol 72*, 9873-9880.

Zufferey, R., Nagy, D., Mandel, R. J., Naldini, L., and Trono, D. (1997). Multiply attenuated lentiviral vector achieves efficient gene delivery in vivo. *Nat Biotechnol 15*, 871-875.

In: Neural Stem Cell Research
Editor: Eric V. Grier, pp. 155-174

ISBN 1-59454-846-3
© 2006 Nova Science Publishers, Inc.

Chapter 7

Classification of Cell Phases in Time-Lapse Images by Vector Quantization and Markov Models

Tuan D. Pham[1,*] **Dat T. Tran**[2,†] **Xiaobo Zhou**[3,‡] **and Stephen T.C. Wong**[4,§]

[1]School of Information Technology, James Cook University
QLD 4811, Australia
[2]School of Information Sciences and Engineering, University of Canberra
ACT 2601, Australia
[3]HCNR Center for Bioinformatics, Harvard Medical School
MA 02215, USA
[4]CNR Center for Bioinformatics, Harvard Medical School
MA 02215, USA

Abstract

Advances in fluorescent probing and microscopic imaging technology provide important tools for biology and medicine research in studying the structures and functions of cells and molecules. Such studies require the processing and analysis of huge amounts of image data, and manual image analysis is very time consuming, thus costly, and also potentially inaccurate and poorly reproducible. Stages of an automated cellular imaging analysis consist of segmentation, feature extraction, classification, and tracking of individual cells in a dynamic cellular population. Image classification of cell phases in a fully automatic manner presents the most difficult task of such analysis. We are interested in applying several advanced computational, probabilistic, and fuzzy-set methods for the computerized classification of cell nuclei in different mitotic phases. We tested several proposed computational procedures with real image sequences recorded over a period of twenty-four hours at every fifteen minutes with a time-lapse fluorescence microscopy. The experimental results have shown that the proposed methods are effective and has potential for higher performance with better cellular feature extraction strategy.

---

[*]E-mail address: tuan.pham@jcu.edu.au, corresponding author
[†]E-mail address: dat.tran@canberra.edu.au
[‡]E-mail address: zhou@crystal.harvard.edu
[§]E-mail address: wong@crystal.harvard.edu

Keywords: fluorescence microscopic imaging, molecular imaging, cell phase identification, vector quantization, k-NN rule, fuzzy c-means, k-means, Markov chain

1 Introduction

High content screening by automated fluorescence microscopy is becoming one of the most widely used research tools to assist scientists in understanding the complex process of cell division or mitosis [1]-[3]. Its power comes from the sensitivity and resolution of automated light microscopy with multi-well plates, combined with the availability of fluorescent probes that are attached to specific subcellular components, such as chromosomes and microtubules, for visualization of cell division or mitosis using standard epi-fluorescence microscopy techniques [4]. By employing a carefully selected reporter probes and filters, fluorescence microscopy allows specific imaging of phenotypes of essentially any cell component [5]. With these probes we can determine both the amount of a cell component, and most critically, its distribution within the cell relative to other components. Typically, 3-4 different components are localized in the same cell using probes that excite at different wavelengths. Any change in cell physiology would cause a redistribution of one or more cellular components, and this redistribution provides a certain cytological marker that allows for scoring of the physiological change.

An essential task for high content screening is to measure cell cycle progression (inter phase, prophase, metaphase, and telophase) in individual cells as a function of time. Cell cycle progress can be identified by measuring nuclear changes.

Automated time-lapse fluorescence microscopy imaging provides an important method for the observation and study of cellular nuclei in a dynamic fashion [6, 7]. Stages of an automated cellular imaging analysis consist of segmentation, feature extraction, classification, and tracking of individual cells in a dynamic cellular population; and the classification of cell phases is considered the most difficult task of such analysis [8].

In time-lapse microcopy images are usually captured in a time interval of more than 10 minutes. During this period dividing nuclei may move far away from each other and daughter cell nuclei may not overlap with their parents. Figure 1 shows the nuclear migration during cell division (two cases of splitting into two); whereas Figure 2 shows the nuclear appearance changes during cell mitosis (top row: split into two; bottom row: split into three). The consecutive image subframes from an image sequence show nuclear size and shape changes during cell mitosis.

Given the advanced fluorescent imaging technology, there still remain technical challenges in processing and analyzing large volumes of images generated by time-lapse microscopy. The increasing quantity and complexity of image data from dynamic microscopy renders manual analysis unreasonably time-consuming. Therefore, automatic techniques for analyzing cell-cycle progress are of considerable interest in the drug discovery process.

Being motivated by the desire to study drug effects on HeLa cells, an ovarian cancer cell line, we applied several computational techniques for identifying individual cell phase changes during a period of time. To extract useful features for the cell-phase identification task, the image segmentation of large image sequences acquired by time-lapse microscopy is necessary. The extracted data can then be used to analyze cell phase changes under drug

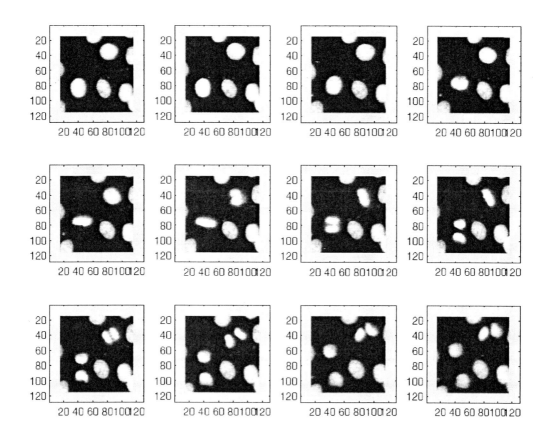

Figure 1: Nuclear migration during cell division.

influence. Segmenting nuclei in time-lapse microscope can be performed by various methods such as thresholding, region growing, or edge detection [9]. Most of these algorithms take into account either the morphological information or the intensity information of the image. Problems may arise when trying to segment touching nuclei because it is very difficult to define the boundary of each individual nuclear. Watershed techniques can be used to segment touching objects [10]. To deal with the over-segmentation problem a post process is needed to merge the fragments. Umesh and Chaudhuri [12] used a connectivity based merging method to merge a tiny cell fragment with a nearby cell if it shares the maximum boundary with that cell. These authors applied their method on a set of 327 cells and a 98% correct segmentation result was reported. This method can only merge small fragments and fails if the size of cell fragments is above a preset value. The bigger fragments are considered as cell by this method. Bleau and Leon [10] used an iterative trial and test approach to merge small regions with their nearby larger regions based on a set of volume, depth, and surface criteria. These authors applied their method to segment the vesicles in live cells; however no experimental results were reported.

   To automate the process of identifying cellular phases using time-lapse fluorescence microscopic image sequences, we first apply a shape-and-size based method which merges

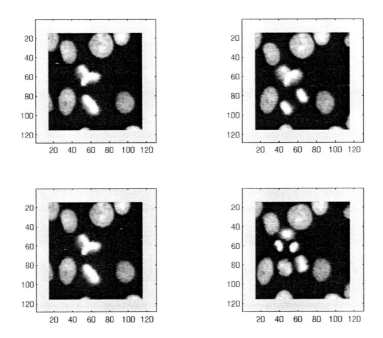

Figure 2: Nuclear appearance changes during cell mitosis.

the over-segmented nuclear fragments. Secondly we extract useful features to discriminate the shapes and intensities of different image cell phases. We then use these image features to train several computational algorithms to identify cancer cells at different phases. The computational methods include the k-NN algorithm; Markov models; and vector quantization method whose various partition designs are based on the k-means, fuzzy c-means, and LBG algorithms.

2   Segmentation of Nuclear Images

Nuclear segmentation is a critical part of the automated analysis system. The segmentation results directly affect the accurate rate of the phase identification. Nuclear images are first segmented and extracted from their background by applying a global thresholding technique, then the watershed technique is used to separate touching nuclei. Finally, a shape-and-size-based procedure was performed to merging the over-segmented nuclear fragments.

2.1   Image thresholding

In time-lapse fluorescence microscopy images of nuclei are bright objects protruding out from a relatively uniform dark background. Thus, they can be segmented by histogram thresholding. In this work the ISODATA algorithm was used to perform image thresholding [13, 14]. By applying the ISODATA technique, an image is initially segmented into two parts using an initial threshold value. The sample mean of the gray values associated with the nuclear pixels and the sample mean of the gray values associated with the background pixels are computed. A new threshold value is then computed as the average of the two sample means. The process is repeated until the change of threshold values reaches convergence.

We found that this algorithm correctly segments most isolated nuclei, but it is unable to segment touching nuclei. The algorithm fails because it assigns the pixels to only two different groups (nuclear and background). If two nuclei are so close and there are no background pixels between them the algorithm will not be able to separate them. We have therefore sought to apply a watershed algorithm to handle this case [8, 15]. We discuss the watershed algorithm in the following subsection.

2.2   Separating touching nuclei

The watershed algorithm first calculates the Euclidean distance map (EDM) of the binary image obtained from the ISODATA algorithm. It then finds the ultimate eroded points (UEP), which are the local maxima of the EDM. The watershed algorithm then dilates each of the UEP as far as possible - either until the edge of the nuclear or the edge of the region of another UEP is reached.

2.3   Fragment merging algorithm

Having discussed that when there is more than one UEP within the same nuclear, the watershed algorithm fails. In such cases the nuclear will be incorrectly divided into several fragments. A fragment merging algorithm is therefore needed to correct such segmentation errors. Nuclei are usually elliptic objects with various shape parameters. In such cases, the compactness can be used to describe the shape of the nuclei. Compactness is defined as the ratio of the square of the perimeter of the nuclear to the area of the nuclear. The value of 1 indicates a circular nuclear. Compactness increases as the contour of the nuclear deviates from the circular shape. If a round nuclear is divided into several fragments, the compactness of each fragment will be larger than the compactness of the entire nuclear. Based on the observation of nuclear shapes and sizes, we have developed a fragment merging technique [13]. This technique can identify over-segmented nuclear fragments and then merges them into single nuclear units. The procedure can be described as follows. Let N be the total number of segmented objects found by the watershed segmentation algorithm. Let T be the minimum size of a nuclear in the image. In this work, a threshold value of 100 pixels is chosen as no single nuclear size is smaller than 100, and larger threshold value will cause small nuclei be identified as fragments and merged with nearby touching nuclei. All touching objects (nuclei) are evaluated and checked. Two objects are considered touching if they belong to the same object in the binary image before the watershed algorithm is applied. This iterative merging process finds the smallest touching objects in each iteration and then uses the checking process to update the segmentation until no more touching objects can be merged. The checking process can be described as follows:

1. If the size of a touching object is less than T it is merged with its smallest touching neighbor.

2. If the size of a touching object is greater than T three compactness values are calculated: the object, touching neighbor of the object, and the two objects as a whole. If the calculated compactness decreases after this merging these two objects are merged.

3   Feature Extraction

After the nuclear segmentation has been performed, it is necessary to perform a morphological closing process on the resulting binary images in order to smooth the nuclear boundaries and fill holes insides the nuclei. These binary images are then used as a mask on applied the original image to arrive at the final segmentation. From this resulting image, features can be extracted. The ultimate goal for feature selection is to assign correct phase to cells via the training of some identification technique. In this work, a set of cell-nuclear features are extracted based on the experience of biologists. To identify the shape and intensity differences between different cell phases, a set of 7 features are extracted. These features include maximum intensity, mean, stand deviation, major axis, minor axis, perimeter, and compactness [8].

Because the feature values have different ranges, the scaling of features is therefore necessary by calculating the z-scores [9]:

$$z_{tk} = \frac{x_{tk} - \bar{m}_k}{s_k} \tag{3.1}$$

where x_{tk} is the k-th feature of the t-th nucleus, $\bar{m}_k$ the mean value of all n cells for feature k, and s_k the mean absolute deviation, that is

$$s_k = \frac{1}{n} \sum_{t=1}^{n} |x_{tk} - \bar{m}_k| \tag{3.2}$$

3.1   Vector quantization

Vector quantization (VQ) is a data reduction method, which is used to convert a feature vector set into a small set of distinct vectors using a clustering technique. Advantages of this reduction are reduced storage and computation. The distinct vectors are called codevectors and the set of codevectors that best represents the training set is called the codebook. Since there is only a finite number of code vectors, the process of choosing the best representation of a given feature vector is equivalent to quantizing the vector and leads to a certain level of quantization error. This error decreases as the size of the codebook increases, however the storage required for a large codebook is non-trivial. The VQ codebook can be used as a model in pattern recognition. The key point of VQ modelling is to derive an optimal codebook which is commonly achieved by using a clustering technique.

3.1.1   VQ procedure

Given a training set of T feature vectors $\mathbf{X} = \{\mathbf{x}_1, \mathbf{x}_2, \ldots, \mathbf{x}_T\}$, where each source vector $\mathbf{x}_t = (x_{t1}, x_{t2}, \ldots, x_{tK})$ is of K dimensions. $\mathbf{C} = \{\mathbf{c}_1, \mathbf{c}_2, \ldots, \mathbf{c}_N\}$ represents the codebook of size N, where $\mathbf{c}_n = (c_{n1}, c_{n2}, \ldots, c_{nk})$, $n = 1, 2, \ldots, N$ are codewords. Each codeword $\mathbf{c}_n$ is assigned to an encoding region R_n in the partition $\Omega = \{R_1, R_2, \ldots, R_N\}$. Then the source vector $\mathbf{x}_t$ can be represented by the encoding region R_n and expressed by

$$V(\mathbf{x}_t) = \mathbf{c}_n, \text{ if } \mathbf{x}_t \in R_n \qquad (3.3)$$

In general, the VQ design can be stated as follows. Given a training set $\mathbf{X}$, the size N of the codebook, we seek to find the codebook $\mathbf{C}$, and the partition Ω such that the average distortion D is minimized. Using the L_2 norm for a squared-error measure, D is defined by

$$D = \frac{1}{TK} \sum_{t=1}^{T} (||\mathbf{x}_t - V(\mathbf{x}_t)||_2)^2 \qquad (3.4)$$

where $||\mathbf{e}_t||_2$ is the L_2 norm or Euclidean norm of the vector $\mathbf{e}_t$ and defined as

$$||\mathbf{e}_t||_2 = (e_{t1}^2 + e_{t2}^2 + \ldots, + e_{tK}^2)^{\frac{1}{2}} \qquad (3.5)$$

Clustering techniques are used to build the codebook $\mathbf{C}$. We review in the subsequent section two non-fuzzy clustering techniques which include k-means and LBG; and two fuzzy clustering techniques which include fuzzy c-means and fuzzy entropy.

3.1.2 k-means partition

Let $U = [u_{nt}]$ be a matrix whose elements are memberships of $\mathbf{x}_t$ in the nth cluster, $n = 1, \ldots, N, t = 1, \ldots, T$. A k-partition space for $\mathbf{X}$ is the matrix U such that [16]

$$u_{nt} \in \{0, 1\} \quad \forall n, t, \qquad \sum_{n=1}^{N} u_{nt} = 1 \quad \forall t, \qquad 0 < \sum_{t=1}^{T} u_{nt} < T \quad \forall n \qquad (3.6)$$

where $u_{nt} = u_n(\mathbf{x}_t)$ is 1 or 0, according to whether $\mathbf{x}_t$ is or is not in the nth cluster, $\sum_{n=1}^{N} u_{nt} = 1 \, \forall t$ means each $\mathbf{x}_t$ is in exactly one of the N clusters, and $0 < \sum_{t=1}^{T} u_{nt} < T$ $\forall n$ means that no cluster is empty and no cluster is all of $\mathbf{X}$ because of $1 < N < T$.

The k-means technique is based on minimization of the sum-of-squared-errors function as follows

$$J(U, \lambda; X) = \sum_{n=1}^{N} \sum_{t=1}^{T} u_{nt} d_{nt}^2 \qquad (3.7)$$

where $U = \{u_{nt}\}$ is a hard k-partition of X, λ is a set of prototypes, in the simplest case, it is the set of cluster centers: $\lambda = \mathbf{C}$, and d_{nt} is the Euclidean norm of $(\mathbf{x}_t - \mathbf{c}_n)$

The k-means algorithm is summarized as follows

1. Given a training data set $\mathbf{X} = \{\mathbf{x}_1, \mathbf{x}_2, \ldots, \mathbf{x}_T\}$, where $\mathbf{x}_t = (x_{t1}, x_{t2}, \ldots, x_{tK})$, $t = 1, 2, \ldots, T$.

2. Initialize membership values $u_{nt}, 1 \leq t \leq T, 1 \leq n \leq N$, at random

3. Given $\epsilon > 0$ (small real number).

4. Set $i = 0$ and $D^{(i)} = 0$. Iteration:

  (a) Compute cluster centers

$$V(\mathbf{x}_t) = \mathbf{c}_n = \sum_{t=1}^{T} u_{nt} \mathbf{x}_t \Big/ \sum_{t=1}^{T} u_{nt} \qquad 1 \le t \le T, 1 \le n \le N \qquad (3.8)$$

  (b) Compute d_{nt} and $D^{(i+1)}$

$$d_{nt} = \|\mathbf{x}_t - V(\mathbf{x}_t)\|_2 \qquad D^{(i+1)} = \frac{1}{TK} \sum_{t=1}^{T} d_{nt}^2 \qquad (3.9)$$

  (c) Update membership values

$$u_{nt} = \begin{cases} 1 & : \quad d_{nt} < d_{jt} \qquad j = 1, \ldots, N, \quad j \ne n \\ 0 & : \quad \text{otherwise} \end{cases} \qquad (3.10)$$

5. Set $D^{(i)} = D^{(i+1)}$ then $i = i + 1$. Go to step (a) if

$$\frac{D^{(i+1)} - D^{(i)}}{D^{(i+1)}} > \epsilon \qquad (3.11)$$

3.1.3   LBG partition

The LBG algorithm [17] requires an initial codebook, and iteratively bi-partitions the code-vectors based on the optimality criteria of nearest-neighbor and centroid conditions until the number of codevectors is reached. It is summarized as follows.

1. Given a training data set $\mathbf{X} = \{\mathbf{x}_1, \mathbf{x}_2, \ldots, \mathbf{x}_T\}$, where $\mathbf{x}_t = (x_{t1}, x_{t2}, \ldots, x_{tK})$, $t = 1, 2, \ldots, T$.

2. Given $\epsilon > 0$ (small real number)

3. Set $N = 1$, compute initial cluster center and average distortion

$$\mathbf{c}_1^* = \frac{1}{T} \sum_{t=1}^{T} \mathbf{x}_t \qquad (3.12)$$

$$D^* = \frac{1}{TK} \sum_{t=1}^{T} (\|\mathbf{x}_t - \mathbf{c}_1^*\|_2)^2 \qquad (3.13)$$

4. Splitting:

$$\begin{aligned} \mathbf{c}_{n1} &= (1 + \epsilon)\mathbf{c}_n^*, \ 1 \le n \le N \\ \mathbf{c}_{n2} &= (1 - \epsilon)\mathbf{c}_n^*, \ 1 \le n \le N \end{aligned}$$

  Set $N = 2N$

5. Set $i = 0$ and let $D^{(i)} = D^*$. Iteration:

    (a) Assign vector to closest codeword

$$V(\mathbf{x}_t) = \mathbf{c}_n^* = \arg\min_n (\|\mathbf{x}_t - \mathbf{c}_n^{(i)}\|_2)^2, \qquad (3.14)$$

$$1 \leq t \leq T, 1 \leq n \leq N$$

    (b) Update cluster centers

$$\mathbf{c}_n^{(i+1)} = \frac{1}{|V(\mathbf{x}_t)|} \sum_{\mathbf{x}_t \in V(\mathbf{x}_t)} \mathbf{x}_t, \ 1 \leq n \leq N \qquad (3.15)$$

    where $|V(\mathbf{x}_t)|$ is the number of $V(\mathbf{x}_t) = \mathbf{c}_n^*$.

    (c) Compute

$$D^{(i+1)} = \frac{1}{TK} \sum_{t=1}^{T} (\|\mathbf{x}_t - V(\mathbf{x}_t)\|_2)^2 \qquad (3.16)$$

    (d) If

$$\frac{D^{(i+1)} - D^{(i)}}{D^{(i+1)}} > \epsilon \qquad (3.17)$$

    then set $i = i + 1$, $D^* = D^{(i)}$, $\mathbf{c}_n^* = \mathbf{c}_n^{(i)}$, $1 \leq n \leq N$, and go to step (a)

6. Repeat steps 4 and 5 until the desired number of codewords is obtained.

3.1.4   Fuzzy c-means partition

Let $U = [u_{nt}]$ be a matrix whose elements are memberships of $\mathbf{x}_t$ in the nth cluster, $n = 1, \ldots, N, t = 1, \ldots, T$. The fuzzy c-partition space for $\mathbf{X}$ is the set of matrices U such that [18]

$$0 \leq u_{nt} \leq 1 \quad \forall n, t, \qquad \sum_{n=1}^{N} u_{nt} = 1 \quad \forall t, \qquad 0 < \sum_{t=1}^{T} u_{nt} < T \quad \forall n$$

$$(3.18)$$

where $0 \leq u_{nt} \leq 1 \ \forall n, t$ means it is possible for each $\mathbf{x}_t$ to have an arbitrary distribution of membership among the N fuzzy clusters.

The FCM technique is based on minimization of the fuzzy squared-errors function [18, 19]

$$J(U, \lambda; \mathbf{X}) = \sum_{n=1}^{N} \sum_{t=1}^{T} u_{nt}^m d_{nt}^2 \qquad (3.19)$$

where $U = \{u_{nt}\}$ is a fuzzy c-partition of $\mathbf{X}$, $m > 1$ is a weighting exponent on each fuzzy membership u_{it} and controls the degree of fuzziness, λ and d_{nt} are defined as in (3.7). The basic idea of the FCM method is to minimize $J(U, \lambda; \mathbf{X})$ over the variables U and λ on the assumption that matrix U, which is part of the optimal pairs for $J(U, \lambda; \mathbf{X})$, identifies the good partition of the data.

The FCM algorithm is summarized as follows.

1. Given a training data set $\mathbf{X} = \{\mathbf{x}_1, \mathbf{x}_2, \ldots, \mathbf{x}_T\}$, where $\mathbf{x}_t = (x_{t1}, x_{t2}, \ldots, x_{tK})$, $t = 1, 2, \ldots, T$.

2. Initialize membership values $u_{nt}, 1 \leq t \leq T, 1 \leq n \leq N$, at random

3. Given $\epsilon > 0$ (small real number).

4. Set $i = 0$ and $D^{(i)} = 0$. Iteration:

   (a) Compute cluster centers

   $$V(\mathbf{x}_t) = \mathbf{c}_n = \sum_{t=1}^{T} u_{nt}^m \mathbf{x}_t \bigg/ \sum_{t=1}^{T} u_{nt}^m \qquad 1 \leq t \leq T, 1 \leq n \leq N \qquad (3.20)$$

   (b) Compute d_{nt} and $D^{(i+1)}$

   $$d_{nt} = \|\mathbf{x}_t - V(\mathbf{x}_t)\|_2 \qquad D^{(i+1)} = \frac{1}{TK} \sum_{t=1}^{T} d_{nt}^2 \qquad (3.21)$$

   (c) Update membership values

   $$u_{nt} = \frac{1}{\sum_{k=1}^{N} \left(d_{nt}^2/d_{kt}^2\right)^{1/(m-1)}} \qquad (3.22)$$

5. Set $D^{(i)} = D^{(i+1)}$ then $i = i + 1$. Go to step (a) if

   $$\frac{D^{(i+1)} - D^{(i)}}{D^{(i+1)}} > \epsilon \qquad (3.23)$$

3.1.5 Fuzzy entropy partition

The fuzzy entropy (FE) technique is based on minimisation of the following function [20]:

$$H(U, \lambda; \mathbf{X}) = \sum_{n=1}^{N}\sum_{t=1}^{T} u_{nt} d_{nt}^2 + m_E \sum_{n=1}^{N}\sum_{t=1}^{T} u_{nt} \log u_{nt} \qquad (3.24)$$

where $U = \{u_{nt}\}$ is a fuzzy c-partition of $\mathbf{X}$ as defined for fuzzy c-means partition, $m_E > 0$ controls the degree of fuzzy entropy, λ and d_{nt} are defined as in (3.19). The basic idea of the FE technique is to minimize $H(U, \lambda; \mathbf{X})$ over the variables U and λ.

The fuzzy entropy algorithm is summarized as follows.

1. Given a training data set $\mathbf{X} = \{\mathbf{x}_1, \mathbf{x}_2, \ldots, \mathbf{x}_T\}$, where $\mathbf{x}_t = (x_{t1}, x_{t2}, \ldots, x_{tK})$, $t = 1, 2, \ldots, T$.

2. Initialize membership values $u_{nt}, 1 \leq t \leq T, 1 \leq n \leq N$, at random

3. Given $\epsilon > 0$ (small real number).

4. Set $i = 0$ and $D^{(i)} = 0$. Iteration:

   (a) Compute cluster centers

   $$V(\mathbf{x}_t) = \mathbf{c}_n = \sum_{t=1}^{T} u_{nt}\mathbf{x}_t \bigg/ \sum_{t=1}^{T} u_{nt} \qquad 1 \le t \le T, 1 \le n \le N \qquad (3.25)$$

   (b) Compute d_{nt} and $D^{(i+1)}$

   $$d_{nt} = \|\mathbf{x}_t - V(\mathbf{x}_t)\|_2 \qquad D^{(i+1)} = \frac{1}{TK}\sum_{t=1}^{T} d_{nt}^2 \qquad (3.26)$$

   (c) Update membership values

   $$\bar{u}_{nt} = \frac{1}{\displaystyle\sum_{k=1}^{N} e^{(d_{nt}^2 - d_{kt}^2)/m_E}} \qquad (3.27)$$

5. Set $D^{(i)} = D^{(i+1)}$ then $i = i + 1$. Go to step (a) if

$$\frac{D^{(i+1)} - D^{(i)}}{D^{(i+1)}} > \epsilon \qquad (3.28)$$

3.1.6   Algorithm for VQ-based cell-phase identification

Given a cell-phase training set $\mathbf{X}^p$, the VQ codebook can be designed for $\mathbf{X}^p$ given N. The identity of this template codebook is then used for identifying an unknown pattern. The training and classification procedures of this VQ-based algorithm are summarized as follows [21].

Training:

1. Given a cell phase set $\mathbf{X}^p$ of phase p: $\mathbf{X}^p \in \mathcal{X}$, where $\mathcal{X}$ is the universe of cell phases.

2. Build a codebook $\mathbf{C}^p$ of N codewords $(\mathbf{c}_1^p, \mathbf{c}_2^p, \ldots, \mathbf{c}_N^p)$ for $\mathbf{X}^p \in \mathbf{Z}$

Identification:

1. Given a cell of an unknown phase $\mathbf{x}$.

2. Calculate the minimum distance between $\mathbf{x}$ and $\mathbf{C}^p, p = 1, \ldots, P$, where P is the number of phases:

$$d_p = \min_n d(\mathbf{x}.\,\mathbf{c}_n^p) \qquad (3.29)$$

   where $d(\cdot)$ is defined in (3.5).

3. Assign $\mathbf{x}$ to phase p that has the minimum distance:

$$p^* = \arg\min_p (d_p) \qquad (3.30)$$

3.2   Markov Modeling

We present herein a Markov-chain modeling method for cell-phase identification. The occurrences of phases in a sequence of cells can be regarded as a stochastic process and hence the cell sequence can be represented as a Markov chain where phases are states. The occurrence of the first phase in the sequence is characterized by the initial probability of the Markov chain and the occurrence of the other phase given the occurrence of its previous phase is characterized by the transition probability. Given a training set of cell sequences, the initial and transition probabilities for Markov chains representing cell sequences are calculated and the set of those probabilities is regarded as a Markov model for that training set.

3.2.1   Concept of Markov modeling

Given a training set of Q sequences $\mathcal{O} = \{\mathcal{O}_1, \mathcal{O}_2, \ldots, \mathcal{O}_Q\}$, each of which is a sequence of T_q random variables $\mathcal{O}_q = \{O_{q1}, O_{q2}, \ldots, O_{qT}\}$. Let $\mathcal{S} = \{s_1, s_2, \ldots, s_M\}$ be the set of M states in a Markov chain. Consider the conditional probabilities

$$Pr(O_{qt} = o_{qt}|O_{q(t-1)} = o_{q(t-1)}, \ldots, O_{q2} = o_{q2}, O_{q1} = o_{q1}) \qquad (3.31)$$

where o_{qt}, $q = 1, 2, \ldots, Q$ and $t = 1, 2, \ldots, T_q$ are values taken by the corresponding variables O_{qt}.

These probabilities are very complicated for calculation, so the Markov assumption is applied to reduce the complexity

$$Pr(O_{qt} = o_{qt}|O_{q(t-1)} = o_{q(t-1)}, \ldots, O_{q2} = o_{q2}, O_{q1} = o_{q1}) = \\ Pr(O_{qt} = o_{qt}|O_{q(t-1)} = o_{q(t-1)}) \qquad (3.32)$$

where $q = 1, 2, \ldots, Q$ and $t = 1, 2, \ldots, T_q$. This means that the event at time t depends only on the immediately preceding event at time $t-1$. The stochastic process based on the Markov assumption is called the Markov process. In order to restrict the variables O_{qt} taking values o_{qt} in the finite set $\mathcal{S}$, the time-invariant assumption is applied

$$Pr(O_{q1} = o_{q1}) = Pr(O_{q1} = s_i) \qquad (3.33)$$

$$Pr(O_{qt} = o_{qt}|O_{q(t-1)} = o_{q(t-1)}) = Pr(O_{qt} = s_j|O_{q(t-1)} = s_i) \qquad (3.34)$$

where $q = 1, 2, \ldots, Q, t = 1, 2, \ldots, T_q, i = 1, , M$ and $j = 1, \ldots, M$. Such the Markov process is called Markov chain.

We now develop a Markov chain-based modeling method to represent phase sequences found in a given set of cells. Define the following parameters

$$\pi = [\pi_i], \qquad \pi_i = Pr(O_{q1} = s_i) \qquad (3.35)$$

$$\mathbf{A} = [a_{ij}], \qquad a_{ij} = Pr(O_{qt} = s_j|O_{q(t-1)} = s_i) \qquad (3.36)$$

where $q = 1, 2, \ldots, Q$, Q is the number of phase sequences, $t = 2, \ldots, T_q$, T_q is the length of the sequence O_q, $i = 1, \ldots, M$ and $j = 1, \ldots, M$, M is the number of phases.

Phases are states in Markov chains and values in the vector π and matrix $\mathbf{A}$ are state initial probabilities and state transition probabilities, respectively. The set $\lambda = (\pi, \mathbf{A})$ is called the Markov phase model that represents the phase sequences in the training cell set as the Markov chains. A method to calculate the model set λ is presented as follows.

The Markov model λ is built to represent the phase sequences, therefore we should find λ such that the probability $Pr(\mathcal{O} = \mathcal{S}|\lambda)$ is maximised. In order to maximise the probability, we first express it as a function of the model λ, then equate its derivative to 0 to find the model set λ.

Using the Markov assumption in (3.32), the probability $Pr(\mathcal{O} = \mathcal{S}|\lambda)$ can be calculated as follows

$$Pr(\mathcal{O} = \mathcal{S}|\lambda) = \prod_{q=1}^{Q} Pr(O_{q1} = o_{q1}|\lambda) \prod_{t=1}^{T_q} Pr(O_{qt} = o_{qt}|O_{q(t-1)} = o_{q(t-1)}, \lambda) \quad (3.37)$$

Applying the time-invariant assumption in (3.33) and (3.34), Eq. (3.37) can be rewritten as follows

$$Pr(\mathcal{O} = \mathcal{S}|\lambda) = \prod_{i=1}^{M} [\pi_i]^{n_i} \prod_{j=1}^{M} [a_{ij}]^{n_{ij}} \quad (3.38)$$

where n_i and n_{ij} are the number of occurrences of $\pi_i = Pr(O_{q1} = s_i)$ and $a_{ij} = Pr(O_{qt} = s_j|O_{q(t-1)} = s_i)$ in the sequence set $\mathcal{O}$, respectively.

In order to take derivatives, the log-probability is used

$$\log Pr(\mathcal{O} = \mathcal{S}|\lambda) = \sum_{i=1}^{M} n_i \log \pi_i + \sum_{i=1}^{M}\sum_{j=1}^{M} n_{ij} \log a_{ij} \quad (3.39)$$

Since the state initial and state transition probabilities have the following property

$$\sum_{i=1}^{M} \pi_i = 1, \qquad \sum_{j=1}^{M} a_{ij} = 1, \qquad i = 1, \ldots, M \quad (3.40)$$

the Lagrange multiplier method is used to maximise the probability $Pr(\mathcal{O} = \mathcal{S}|\lambda)$. Consider the following Lagrangian

$$L = \sum_{i=1}^{M} n_i \log \pi_i + a\left[\sum_{i=1}^{M} \pi_i - 1\right] + \sum_{i=1}^{M}\sum_{j=1}^{M} n_{ij} \log a_{ij} + \sum_{i=1}^{M} b_i\left[\sum_{j=1}^{M} a_{ij} - 1\right] \quad (3.41)$$

After equating derivatives of L over π_k and a_{ik} to 0 and solving those equations, we obtain

$$\pi_i = \frac{n_i}{\displaystyle\sum_{k=1}^{M} n_k}, \qquad a_{ij} = \frac{n_{ij}}{\displaystyle\sum_{k=1}^{M} n_{ik}} \tag{3.42}$$

3.3 VQ-Markov Modeling

Given a cell-phase training set X^p, a VQ codebook can be designed for X^p given N. The identity of this template codebook is then used for identifying an unknown pattern. The training and classification procedures of this VQ-Markov algorithm are summarized as follows.

Training:

1. Given $\mathcal{X}$ as the universe of cell phases.

2. Train VQ-based phase models

   (a) Divide the set $\mathcal{X}$ into P distinct subsets $\mathbf{X}^1, \mathbf{X}^2, \ldots, \mathbf{X}^P$, where each $\mathbf{X}^p$ contains cells of phase p.

   (b) For each subset $\mathbf{X}^p$, train a VQ-based phase model using the training algorithm in Section 3.1.6

3. Train Markov model for all phases

   (a) Align cells in the set $\mathcal{X}$ as sequences of cells

   (b) Extract Q phase sequences $\mathcal{O}_1, \mathcal{O}_2, \ldots, \mathcal{O}_Q$ from the set $\mathcal{X}$

   (c) Using Q phase sequences, calculate π and $\mathbf{A}$ according to (3.42)

Identification:

1. Given an unknown sequence of cells $\mathbf{X} = \{\mathbf{x}_1, \mathbf{x}_2, \ldots, \mathbf{x}_T\}$.

2. Identify phase for the first cell $\mathbf{x}_1$ in the sequence as follows

   (a) Calculate the minimum distance between $\mathbf{x}_1$ and $\mathbf{C}^p$, $p = 1, \ldots, P$, where P is the number of phases:
   $$d_p = \min_n d(\mathbf{x}_1, \mathbf{c}_n^p) \tag{3.43}$$
   where $d(\cdot)$ is defined in (3.5).

   (b) Calculate the similarity score $S(\mathbf{x}_1, p)$

   $$S(\mathbf{x_1}, p) = \frac{\pi_p}{\displaystyle\sum_{k=1}^{P} \left(d_p/d_k\right)^{1/(m-1)}} \tag{3.44}$$

   where $m > 1$.

(c) Assign $\mathbf{x}_1$ to the phase p^* that has the maximum score:

$$p^* = \arg\max_p S(\mathbf{x}_1, p) \tag{3.45}$$

3. For each cell $\mathbf{x}_i$, $i = 2, \ldots, T$, identify it as follows

(a) Calculate the minimum distance between $\mathbf{x}_i$ and $\mathbf{C}^p$, $p = 1, \ldots, P$, where P is the number of phases:

$$d_p = \min_n d(\mathbf{x}_i, \mathbf{c}_n^p) \tag{3.46}$$

where $d(\cdot)$ is defined in (3.5).

(b) Calculate the similarity score $S(\mathbf{x}_i, p)$

$$S(\mathbf{x}_i, p) = \frac{a_{p^*p}}{\sum_{k=1}^{P} (d_p/d_k)^{1/(m-1)}} \tag{3.47}$$

where $m > 1$ and p^* is the identified phase of the previous cell.

(c) Assign $\mathbf{x}_i$ to the phase p^* that has the maximum score:

$$p^* = \arg\max_p S(\mathbf{x}_i, p) \tag{3.48}$$

4 Experimental Results

Four nuclear sequences were provided by the Department of Cell Biology at the Harvard Medical School to test the efficiency of the proposed system. Imaging was performed by time-lapse fluorescence microscopy with a time interval of 15 minutes. Two types of sequences were used denoting drug treated and untreated. Cell cycle progress was affected by drug and some or all of the cells in the treated sequences were arrested in metaphase. Cell cycle progress in the untreated sequences was not affected. Cells without drug treatment will usually undergo one division during this period of time.

Seven features extracted for each cell are considered as the feature vectors for training and testing several identification approaches including the k-NN algorithm;

Table 1. Cell-phase identification rate

Computational model	Identification rate (%)
k-NN	82.04
k-means	85.25
k-means and Markov	86.65
LBG-VQ	85.54
LBG-VQ and Markov	86.61
FE-VQ	86.13
FE-VQ and Markov	87.32
FCM-VQ	88.24
FCM-VQ and Markov	88.35

VQ approaches based on the k-means, fuzzy c-means (FCM), fuzzy entropy (FE), LBG algorithms, and the combinations of VQ and Markov models. The parameter k was set to be 6 for the k-NN algorithm [9]. The degree of fuzziness m and degree of fuzzy entropy m_F were set to be 1.1 and 0.05, respectively.

There are 5 phases to be identified: interphase, prophase, metaphase, anaphase, and arrested metaphase. We divided the data set into 5 subsets for training 5 models and a subset for identification. Each of the 5 training sets for 5 phases contains 5000 cells, which were extracted from the cell sequences labeled from 590 to 892. These sequences were also used to calculate the Markov models. The identification set contains sequences labeled from 1 to 589. There are 249,547 cells in this identification set.

The identification results obtained from 9 computational models are presented in Table 1. It can be seen that the combination of the FCM and Markov models yields the best performance (88.35%), which outperformed the k-NN by more than 6%. The experimental results can be generally noted that the probabilistic modeling of the VQ code vectors by Markov chains always increases the identification rates in all VQ partitioning strategies being either k-means, fuzzy c-means, fuzzy entropy, or LBG algorithms. Moreover, the computational time for any of the VQ methods was significantly less than that for the k-NN method, particularly when the value for k of the k-NN rule increases.

5   Concluding Remarks

Several computational techniques for the identification of cell phases using time-lapse fluorescence microscopic image sequences that we have discussed are methods for pattern classification. In general, pattern recognition methods have been applied for solving many important practical problems which can be either abstract (conceptual classification) or concrete (physical classification). Methodologies and techniques for machine learning and recognition have been extensively studied by many researchers from many different disciplines. However, there is still no unifying theory that can be applied to all kinds of pattern recognition problems. Most techniques for pattern classification and recognition are problem-oriented. Among many approaches for pattern classification including linear discriminant analysis, Bayesian classifier, Markov chains, hidden Markov models, neural networks, and support vector machines, the k-NN decision rule, which is a procedure for deciding the membership of an unknown sample by a majority vote of the k-nearest neighbors, is one of the most popular classification methods chosen for solving many practical problems in many disciplines ranging from image, text, speech, to life and natural sciences [22]-[27].

Although the k-NN rule is a suboptimal procedure, it has been shown that with unlimited number of samples the error rate for the 1-NN rule is not more than twice the optimal Bayes error rate [16], and as k increases this error rate asymptotically approaches the optimal rate [28]. Given the advantages of the k-NN classifier, it has been pointed out that the assumption of equal weights in the assignment of an input vector to class labels can reduce the accuracy of the k-NN algorithm, particularly when there is a strong degree of overlap between the sample vectors [29, 30]. This is a problem for the application of the k-NN rule for the identification of cell phases in this study, whose identification rate is lowest among other methods (82.04%). One strategy to overcome this problem encountered by the k-NN algorithm is the use of fuzzy k-NN algorithms [29, 30] which assigns a fuzzy membership for an unknown sample to class label as a linear combination of the fuzzy membership grades of k nearest samples. After the assignment of the fuzzy membership grades of an unknown vector to all class labels, the fuzzy k-NN classifier assigns the unknown sample to the class label whose fuzzy membership for that class is maximum.

The incorporation of probabilistic analysis using Markov chains into the template matching using vector quantization approach helps improve the identification rates with various clustering criterion (k-means, fuzzy c-means, and LBG algorithms). From the experimental results, it can be seen that the fuzzy vector quantization (either fuzzy entropy or fuzzy c-means) is superior to either the k-means or LBG based vector quantization methods. The FCM algorithm seeks to partition a data set into a specified number of fuzzy regions which are represented by the corresponding fuzzy prototypes. The degrees of each cellular-image feature vector that belong to different clusters are characterized by the corresponding fuzzy membership grades taking real values between 0 and 1. Thus, the use of the fuzzy c-means algorithm provides more effective analysis of the present problem where the image boundaries of different classes are vaguely defined.

Vector quantization (VQ) is an approach that has been widely used in speech and image processing for data reduction by building a codebook of distinct vectors that represent a very large collection of raw vectors. Despite its advantages, VQ suffers from an inherent distortion in representing an actual analysis vector. As the size of the codebook increases, the size of the quantization error decreases. However, with any codebook there always exists some level of quantization error. So when vector quantization is implemented for Markov models (MMs), VQ-based MMs have two kinds of error: quantization error caused by the quantized input vectors, and estimation error caused by estimating the occurrence probabilities of clusters in each MM state. Therefore Markov models based on fuzzy vector quantization is an improved approach which is designed to reduce those errors.

The selection of useful features is a very important task for any classifier. In this work we have selected seven features of the nuclear images to train several classifiers which are all superior to the k-NN decision rule. However, the issue of feature selection is worth investigating in our future research as new useful image features can certainly enhance the performance of the proposed classifiers, particularly the FCM-VQ Markov-chain based classifier which has achieved the highest identification rate.

Molecular imaging is an exciting area of research in life sciences, which provides an outstanding tool for the study of diseases at the molecular or cellular levels. Some molecular imaging techniques have been implemented for clinical applications [31]. To contribute to this emerging imaging technology, we have presented and discussed several computational models for the identification of cellular phases based on fluorescent imaging data. This task is an important component for any computerized imaging system which automates the screening of high-content, high-throughput fluorescent images of mitotic cells to aid biomedical or biological researchers to study the mitotic data at dynamic ranges for various applications including the study of the complexity of cell processes, and the screening of novel anti-mitotic drugs as potential cancer therapeutic agents.

Acknowledgments

The time-lapse fluorescence microscopic image data set was provided by our collaborator, Dr. Randy King of the Department of Cell Biology, Harvard Medical School. Research grants from the HCNR-CBI program and NIH-NLM R01 LM008696-01 to Dr. Stephen Wong are also acknowledged.

References

[1] Fox, S., Accommodating cells in HTS, *Drug Discovery World*, **5** (2003) 21-30.

[2] Feng, Y., Practicing cell morphology based screen, *European Pharmaceutical Review*, **7** (2002) 7-11.

[3] Dunkle, R., Role of image informatics in accelerating drug discovery and development, *Drug Discovery World*, **5** (2003) 75-82.

[4] Yarrow, J.C., et al., Phenotypic screening of small molecule libraries by high throughput cell imaging, *Comb Chem High Throughput Screen*, **6** (2003) 279-286.

[5] Murphy, D.B., *Fundamentals of light Microscopy and Electronic Imaging*. Wiley-Liss, 2001.

[6] Hiraoka, Y., and Haraguchi, T., Fluorescence imaging of mammalian living cells, *Chromosome Res*, **4** (1996) 173-176.

[7] Kanda, T., Sullivan, K. F., and Wahl G. M., Histone-GFP fusion protein enables sensitive analysis of chromosome dynamics in living mammalian cells, *Current Biology*, **8** (1998) 377-85.

[8] Chen, X., Zhou, X., and Wong, S.T.C., Automated segmentation, classification, and tracking cancer cell nuclei in time-lapse microscopy, *IEEE Trans. on Biomedical Engineering*, in press.

[9] MacAulay, C., and Palcic, B. A., comparison of some quick and simple threshold selection methods for stained cells, *Anal. Quant. Cytol. Histol.*, **10** (1988) 134-138.

[10] Bleau A., and Leon J.L., Watershed-based segmentation and region merging, *Computer Vision and Image Understanding*, **77** (2000) 317-370.

[11] Paliwal, K.K. and Rao, P.V.S., Application of k-nearest-neighbor decision rule in vowel recognition. *IEEE Trans. Pattern Analysis and Machine Intelligence*, **5** (1983) 229-231.

[12] Umesh, A.P.S., and Chaudhuri B.B., An efficient method based on watershed and rule-based merging for segmentation of 3-D histopathological images, *Pattern Recognition*, **34** (2001) 1449-1458.

[13] Norberto M., Andres S., Carlos Ortiz S. Juan Jose V., Francisco P., and Jose Miguel G., Applying watershed algorithms to the segmentation of clustered nuclei, *Cytometry*, **28** (1997) 289-297.